Praise for
Growing Trees and Shrubs Indoors

D. J. Herda brings all his talents as a writer and his personal experiences as a gardener to bear in this fascinating, encyclopedic compendium dealing with the nature and care of trees and shrubs. It would not surprise me to learn that many readers of this book might later choose to turn the interiors of their once barren homes into lush forests and woodlands. My guess is that any lover of nature would enjoy owning this book.

— Arnold M. Ludwig, author, *The Price of Greatness* and *King of the Mountain*

This is a great read! If, like me, you think plants are just decorations, think again. D.J. explains that they are much, much more than that. Just reading the preface transformed my understanding of, and respect for, indoor plants. As a behavioural psychologist, I am well aware of the benefits plants can have on our minds, but I was less aware of the impact they have on our health. In summary, this book is an enlightening journey through the world of indoor plants. Clearly written and beautifully illustrated. Even if you don't have any interest in indoor plants you should definitely read *Growing Trees and Shrubs Indoors*. It's a real eye-opener!

— Phillip Adcock, commercial psychologist, and author, *Master Your Brain*

D.J. Herda's book is a comprehensive view into not only how to grow trees and shrubs in your home or office, but also why. Sure, many of us know the health advantages of having indoor plants — air purification, better productivity, and an increase in overall mood — yet we generally don't look beyond buying the basic houseplants. D.J. explains the benefits of going big and then tells us how to do it, from what kinds of trees to buy to how to take care of them. He covers everything from watering needs and light requirements to propagation to keep costs down, all in an effort to help you create a verdant home that has the health benefits of being outside.

— Deanna Duke, author, *The Non-Toxic Avenger*

When I was young (I am 72 years old now) I tried growing a couple of dwarf shrubs inside my apartment. It only took a couple of weeks before the leaves turned yellow, and eventually the plant died. If I only knew then what I have learned from D. J. Herda's new book, I would have been called "Dr. Green Thumb" instead of "Dr. Death." And who would have thought that these trees and shrubs could improve my health as well as the health of my home environment? Well-written, entertaining, and loaded with useful information!

— Dr. Al Danenberg, periodontist, Certified Functional Medicine Practitioner, Certified Primal Health Coach

This book explains which plants are the most beneficial for a healthy indoor environment and how to use these natural "air purifiers" so that they are attractive and thriving contributors to any household. The author distills a lifetime of plant experience into easy-to-follow instruction on how to select, combine, shape, and maintain indoor trees and shrubs, giving an amateur like me the confidence to green my home for health. The annotated list, complete with photos, is especially helpful to those of us who can't remember plant names and don't speak Latin.

— Paula Baker-LaPorte, FAIA, BBNC, and co-author, *Prescriptions for a Healthy House*

GROWING
Trees & Shrubs
INDOORS

BREATHE NEW LIFE INTO YOUR HOME
WITH LARGE PLANTS

D.J. HERDA

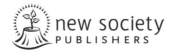
new society
PUBLISHERS

Cover design by Diane McIntosh.

Cover photo: © iStock
Background image: © AdobeStock_90796513

Printed in Canada. First printing October 2019.

Inquiries regarding requests to reprint all or part of *Growing Trees and Shrubs Indoors* should be addressed to New Society Publishers at the address below. To order directly from the publishers, please call toll-free (North America) 1-800-567-6772, or order online at www.newsociety.com

Any other inquiries can be directed by mail to:
New Society Publishers
P.O. Box 189, Gabriola Island, BC V0R 1X0, Canada
(250) 247-9737

LIBRARY AND ARCHIVES CANADA CATALOGUING IN PUBLICATION
Title: Growing trees & shrubs indoors : breathe new life into your home with large plants /
    D.J. Herda.
Other titles: Growing trees and shrubs indoors
Names: Herda, D. J., 1948- author.
Description: Includes bibliographical references and index.
Identifiers: Canadiana (print) 20190133384 | Canadiana (ebook) 20190133392 |
    ISBN 9780865719125 (softcover) | ISBN 9781550927054 (PDF) |
    ISBN 9781771423014 (EPUB)
Subjects: LCSH: Trees. | LCSH: Shrubs. | LCSH: House plants. | LCSH: Indoor gardening.
    | LCSH: Indoor air pollution—Prevention.
Classification: LCC SB435.5 .H47 2019 | DDC 635.9/65—dc23

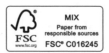 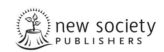

Funded by the Government of Canada | Financé par le gouvernement du Canada | Canada

New Society Publishers' mission is to publish books that contribute in fundamental ways to building an ecologically sustainable and just society, and to do so with the least possible impact on the environment, in a manner that models this vision.

Contents

Preface

TREES AND SHRUBS. Dozens of them. Thousands. Millions. Trillions! They dominate the landscape in all four corners of the world. They adapt to the harshest climates and the most grueling conditions. They generate oxygen and remove carbon dioxide from the atmosphere around us. They provide shade in the summer and a windbreak in the winter. They cut heating and cooling costs for our homes. They may even produce beautiful, aromatic flowers and edible, healthful fruit and nuts!

But why on Earth would anyone want to grow trees and shrubs indoors? They are, after all, the mega-monsters of the plant world. They're huge and gobble up tons of space. They're difficult to grow under the best of conditions. And they're nearly impossible to move around.

Or are they?

Actually, trees and shrubs make great indoor companions for human domiciles. They are masters of environmental cleansing, which is extraordinarily good news since numerous studies show that the most polluted air we breathe comes from inside our own homes — not out. The EPA estimates that indoor pollution levels are between two-to-five times higher than they are outside. Some of the specific pollutants you breathe in can be as much as 100 times more concentrated indoors!

Both the National Cancer Institute (NCI) and the Centers for Disease Control and Prevention (CDC) have established that 80 percent of all cancers may be attributed to factors not from your genetic makeup or your diet but from your environment. The sources of indoor pollution are a combination of interactions between buildings, their occupants, the climate, construction materials, furnishings, and specific contaminants. Among the causes are hundreds of different harmful volatile organic compounds (VOCs) that are your home's usual suspects. These include asbestos, bacteria, viruses, building materials, painting and decorating products, carbon monoxide, carpets, cleaning supplies and household chemicals, cockroaches, dust mites, dust, formaldehyde, lead, pet dander, radon, secondhand smoke, fire retardants, and other miscellany.

VOCs are a specific and dangerous type of pollution emitted from the use of everyday products such as aerosol sprays, cleaning supplies, wood preservatives, hobby supplies, and pressed wood products commonly used in furniture and building materials. Some of the more familiar names of these VOCs are benzene, formaldehyde, xylene, and toluene.

Scary? Only to the uninitiated. Recent studies have shown that potted plants improve your work and living spaces by reducing your blood pressure, increasing your attention span and productivity, lowering your anxiety levels, and reducing the chance for stroke and heart attack.

Other research has demonstrated that working around plants leads to a higher degree of accuracy and better results in performance. Memory retention and concentration also improve by an average of 20 percent.

While most leafy plants are adept at removing some pollution from your indoor air, scientists have discovered several that are better at removing VOCs than others. NASA was behind some of the initial research in 1989 to unearth specific plants that might be useful to reduce pollution in sealed environments — such as in space capsules and the space station. Their study showed that some indoor plants removed as much as 87 percent of all airborne pollutants!

Researchers have identified the following houseplants as those that are most beneficial at removing targeted VOCs.

- **Jade plant:** Particularly good at absorbing toluene emitted from gasoline, paint, kerosene, and lacquers.
- **Spider plant:** Excellent for absorbing up to 90 percent of formaldehyde and carbon monoxide from tobacco smoke, O-xylene from fuels, and P-xylene in plastics.
- **Scarlet start:** In the Bromeliad family (pineapples), this plant purifies the air of 90 percent of benzenes emitted from glues, furniture wax, detergent, and paint.
- **Caribbean tree cactus:** This plant can absorb up to 80 percent of the ethylbenzene wherever it's grown. Ethylbenzene is an emission from electronic products, construction materials, garden-care products, toys, and furniture.
- **Dracaena:** This stunning all-green or variegated-leaf plant absorbs 90 percent

of the acetone from household cleaners and nail polish remover.

- **Fern:** The delicate fronts remove numerous pollutants from the air while providing healthful humidity for your environment.
- **Peace lily:** In either solid or variegated-leaf variety, it blooms in the spring and absorbs electromagnetic radiation from digital devices while it humidifies the air.
- **English ivy:** An excellent companion plant for trees and shrubs, it's useful in absorbing the toxins from cigarette smoke and cleansing the air for asthma sufferers.
- **Ficus:** Slightly more challenging to care for, the Ficus cleanses odors from the air and reduces toxic substances from both home and office.
- **Snake plant** (Mother-in-law's tongue): Another excellent companion plant, this is easy to care for and cleanses the air of benzene and formaldehyde while increasing the room's oxygen content while you sleep.
- **Philodendron and pathos:** These companion plants are easily grown and look great hanging over the sides of pots. They efficiently detoxify formaldehyde.
- **Bamboo palm:** Also known as the reed palm, this tree thrives indoors and readily absorbs formaldehyde outgasses from furniture.

How Much Is Enough?

NASA researchers suggest you use at least one potted plant per 100 square feet of home or office space for maximum air-purifying effects. That distills down to one large plant or several smaller ones for a spacious area such as a typical family room or a master bedroom en suite.

It's true that trees and shrubs can take up a lot of space, but they don't have to. Many species and hybrid varieties are compact enough for small to medium-sized pots. Others, while growing tall, can utilize all that indoor "dead space" above our heads — especially in foyers, stairwells, and homes with open floor plans and cathedral ceilings.

And when it comes time to move your large plants around, you'll find doing so a cinch using a trivet on casters. Placed beneath even the largest of pots, trivets make relocating indoor trees and shrubs from one place to another easier.

How do I know? I've been growing trees and shrubs indoors for the better part of three decades. I wouldn't dream of living anywhere that didn't boast a dozen or more of these foliar monsters sharing my family's space. Plants make us feel good, bring a piece of the outdoors in, cleanse and oxygenate the air we breathe, create dramatic decorating details, and change — some of them — with the seasons. As a bonus, they help increase your cognitive reasoning, stretch your memory, and kick your immune system up a notch or two. (I haven't had the flu or even a common cold in more than a dozen years now. Knock on *Ficus benjamina*!)

The sheer size and beauty of trees and shrubs create an efficient window screen that helps keep the blinding rays of the sun out of our eyes when we're watching TV or working at our computers. They prevent our furniture from fading or rotting from the sun's damaging rays. And, so far as the dramatic effect on your décor, forget that end table and lamp. Bring in a *Dracaena marginata*, *Schefflera*, or a Norfolk Island pine, instead.

If you're worried about your trees and shrubs outgrowing your home or apartment, well, you can give up that ghost, too. Utilizing two simple techniques called "pruning" and "heading back," you can keep nearly any botanical specimen precisely the size you want — year after year — both in height and girth.

But the number one advantage to growing trees and shrubs indoors is the number one reason behind nearly everything we do in life.

Health

Being near so many large plants is not only physically healthful but also emotionally stimulating, calming, soothing, and sedating. (Yes, all of that.) In fact, large plants are so beneficial to humans from a health standpoint that specialized cutting-edge hospital and medical facility design teams are incorporating them into their fundamental architectural concepts. Institutional designers have learned that walls of fiddle-leaf fig trees in a hospital environment, for example, cut down on sound pollution while contributing to shorter hospital stays and fewer medical complications for their patients, resulting in lower patient costs.

One of the reasons is that large plants produce a radical change in the molecular structure of the air around them — and us! — for the better; and, since most people spend far more time inside than out, it makes sense to surround ourselves with these miracles of molecular transmogrification.

Trees and shrubs offer yet another healthful benefit that has only recently come to light: they act as some of the world's most efficient and effective humidifiers, turning the driest and least healthy of rooms into the most hospitable of human habitats. As a bonus, they produce none of the potentially deadly pathogens of costly conventional humidification systems!

And that's only the beginning.

At the Landscaping and Human Health Laboratory in Champagne-Urbana, Illinois, researchers are hard at work developing the best strategies for impacting human health and happiness. They concentrate on trees and shrubs in and around the home to increase positive mental attitude (PMA) and to reduce human aggression. They have uncovered how rational planting can strengthen the welfare of the community and enhance the individual's ability to cope with various physical and mental diseases and illnesses via increased immunity, vitality, attention span, self-control, and capacity for learning.

At the same time, new studies are showing how trees and shrubs in the home environment can significantly reduce Attention-Deficit/Hyperactivity Disorder (ADHD) and other human diseases. Several studies suggest that trees and shrubs in the home reduce the incidence and severity of domestic violence.[1]

Studies conducted at the Rodale Institute, the Plants for Human Health Institute, the University of Minnesota's Healthy Plants-Healthy Lives Institute, NC State University's Plants for Human Health Institute, and other research facilities are also yielding promising findings with the correlation of trees and shrubs to human wellness. Not only in the home but also in schools, churches, and workplaces.

So, if you're looking for a single word that sums up all of the reasons for growing trees and shrubs indoors, sorry. This book can't help you. But if you're looking for the most important reason for growing these age-old wonders of the plant world inside your home, I can sum it up in a few simple words: For your health!

Science Says

The vast majority of plants absorb carbon dioxide (CO_2) at night and give off oxygen (O_2) during the day. But a few plants work a little differently, both absorbing CO_2 and giving off O_2 at night. That makes them especially beneficial in sleeping areas, where reducing carbon dioxide and increasing oxygen levels results in a deeper, healthier, more restful sleep.

The scientific explanation behind this wondrous phenomenon is relatively simple, if you're a plant. Otherwise, suffice to say that the plants listed below perform a type of photosynthesis called crassulacean acid metabolism (CAM).

There are two means by which plants generate photosynthesis. One is by light reaction, meaning O_2 is released by splitting H_2O (water) molecules into hydrogen and oxygen. The other means is by dark reaction (Calvin cycle) in which plants use CO_2 to make sugars to drive the process of photosynthesis.

The energy behind both these reactions comes from sunlight. CO_2 is absorbed via the plant's stomata, and O_2 is released in the same channels. In CAM photosynthesis metabolism, the plant opens the stomata at night to minimize water loss and keeps it closed during the day to conserve life-sustaining water.

The bottom line is that, if you want to pop out of bed reinvigorated and ready to tackle the problems of the day, include one or more of these plants in your bedroom:

- **Areca palm:** These are slow-to-moderate growers in sun or shade and can reach heights of 15 to 20 feet outdoors. They're wide at the top, so they make excellent finely textured specimens if given enough room.
- **Neem tree:** Synonymous with numerous health benefits, neem trees also purify the air during nighttime by emitting oxygen. Superstition calls for the trees to be planted inside the house, especially in the center or courtyard of the house, and that belief is scientifically true since neem acts as a natural pesticide.
- **Snake plant:** Much like aloe vera, snake plants also emit oxygen at night. So, get one in your house and breathe in a healthy environment even during the night.

- **Aloe vera:** Whenever a list of plants with benefits is made, aloe vera tops the charts *always*. Listed as one of the plants improving the air of NASA, aloe vera emits oxygen at night and increases the longevity of your life. It's practically a no-maintenance plant that adds an elegant touch of beauty to any room.
- **Gerber daisy:** Beautiful daisy-like plants, these make good companions for numerous trees and shrubs while brightening up any room.
- **Christmas cactus:** Long-blooming companion plants or small shrubs, these can get quite dramatic with their everlasting blossoms of red, pink, or white.
- **Tulsi:** Also known as holy basil, this plant is widely used for its medicinal qualities and makes an excellent companion plant for trees and shrubs.
- **Peepal tree:** Despite the superstition that spirits dwell within this tree, peepals have several benefits that make them rather important plants in their native lands. They not only emit oxygen at night but also are useful in controlling diabetes and treating constipation and asthma.
- **Orchid:** Beautiful and beneficial, orchids are the perfect choice for a brightly lit corner of your bedroom. Apart from emitting oxygen during the nighttime, orchids also clean the air of xylene, a potent pollutant found in paints, while filling the room with their exotic tropical fragrance.

Making Complex Simple

Interestingly, oxygen emitted by plants is a waste product from the plant's process of photosynthesis, which uses energy from the sun (or a compatible daylight-balanced, full-spectrum artificial light source) to turn carbon dioxide (CO_2) and water (H_2O) into sugar ($C_6H_{12}O_6$), giving off oxygen (O_2) as a by-product. That's *photosynthesis.*

Plants also break down sugar ($C_6H_{12}O_6$) into carbon dioxide (CO_2) and water (H_2O), but they need oxygen (O_2) to do so. That's *cellular respiration.*[2]

Whatever the process, you'll want to move some of these plants into your bedroom for a better night's sleep!

If that's not good enough news for your tired ears, scientists say they have succeeded in genetically modifying a common houseplant so that it improves air quality. Researchers from the University of Washington (UW) have genetically altered pothos ivy (*Epipremnum aureum*) to remove chloroform and benzene from the air surrounding it.

The plants have been modified so they express a mammalian protein, called 2E1, which enables them to transfer the harmful pollutants into compounds that can support plant growth. Since the insides of our homes can contain small molecules such as chloroform or benzene (a component of gasoline) from boiling water, storing cars and lawnmowers in attached garages, and even simple showering, they could benefit from "super-cleansers."

Tiny Toxic Molecules Too Small for HEPA

Many of the airborne pollutants in our homes are too small to be captured by even HEPA air filters. That creates a problem in that long-term exposure to these microscopic pollutants has been linked to cancer.

"People haven't really been talking about these hazardous organic compounds in homes, and I think that's because we couldn't do anything about them," according to senior study investigator Stuart Strand, a research professor in the UW's civil and environmental engineering department. "Now we've engineered houseplants to remove these pollutants for us."[3]

The scientists got their inspiration from nature by focusing on a protein called cytochrome P450 2E1, or 2E1 for short. The 2E1 protein is naturally present in all mammals, including humans. In our bodies, 2E1 turns benzene into a chemical called phenol, and chloroform into carbon dioxide and chloride ions.

Unfortunately, the protein is located in our liver and not available to battle air pollution. That's where Strand's team came in. "We decided we should have this reaction occur outside of the body in a plant, an example of the 'green liver' concept," he explained. "And 2E1 can be beneficial for the plant, too. Plants use carbon dioxide and chloride ions to make their food, and they use phenol to help make components of their cell walls."[4]

So, researchers developed a synthetic version of the gene and, through slow, methodic measures, eventually introduced it to the pothos so that every cell in the plant expressed the protein. They then tested their new GMO plants by taking both a non-modified and a modified plant and putting them in glass tubes filled with either benzene or chloroform gas.

The concentration of each pollutant in each tube was tracked over the next 11 days. The levels did not change at all for the unmodified plants; the modified plants, though, showed the concentration of chloroform had dropped by 82% after only 3 days. By day 6, the chloroform was nearly undetectable. The level of benzene also decreased in the modified plant vials, although at the slower rate of a 75% decrease over an eight-day span.[5]

The team believes the plants will work inside homes, but they would need good airflow or a fan aimed directly at the plants for maximum effectiveness. "If you had a plant growing in the corner of a room," Strand says, "it will have some effect on that room, but without airflow, it will take a long time for a molecule at the other end of the house to reach the plant."

Bolstered by the success of their experiments, Strand's researchers are now attempting to develop modifications for other common household pollutants, including formaldehyde, wood smoke, and furniture.

Could researchers one day turn air pollution into a thing of the past simply by changing a few genetic elements of various hardy plants?

In the words of the immortal physicist Albert Einstein, "Why not?"

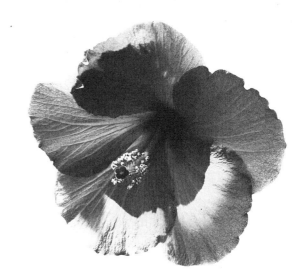

Chapter One:

Why Trees and Shrubs?

I F YOU ROOT AROUND THE SHELVES of your neighborhood bookstore long enough, do you know what you'll find? Dust! And books, too, of course. Plenty of books dedicated to growing all sorts of indoor plants. Flowering plants. Small houseplants. Cacti. Succulents. Bromeliads. Even fruits and vegetables. So why another book — and why about trees and shrubs?

Well, if you've ever gone outside in the spring, opened up a spadeful of earth, inserted a young sapling, and heeled the hole closed again, you know why. Even if you have a massive yard filled with beautiful flowers and bushy shrubs, there's a special thrill all of its own in planting a young tree. The pleasure comes partly, I suppose, from the anticipation of knowing that a tree 2 feet tall today will be 4 feet tall tomorrow — then 6 feet, 10 feet, 90 feet, and more. You have played a role in creating one of the most amazing things in nature. Long after you've gone and your relatives have forgotten how little you bequeathed them in your will, the tree you planted will remain for the benefit of mankind, checking destructive erosion, screening out the sun's scorching rays, drawing impurities from the air, and replacing pollutants with life-giving oxygen and humidity.

Can you imagine what our existence on Earth would be if there were no trees? Our little planet would quickly dry up and crumble away. No living thing could survive. We would all perish.

For centuries now, man has turned toward the heavens to view nature's most miraculous living creations — spiraling, majestic towers of wood and living cells. Our earliest ancestors looked upon trees with both awe and wonder. There was life in these creations … and longevity. If man was not struck by the complexity of the other components of life around him, he was humbled by the trees that existed long before he came and would last long after his passing from the Earth.

> I remember, I remember,
> The roses, red and white,
> The vi'lets, and the lily-cups,
> Those flowers made of light!
> The lilacs where the robin built,
> And where my brother set
> The laburnum on his birthday, —
> The tree is living yet!
>
> Thomas Hood, "I Remember"

Trees are not the oldest form of plants on Earth. From the vast seas that gave birth to evolution came the algae and bacteria; they were eventually followed by the more recognizable plant life — mosses and ferns. Even so, trees have been around for 300 million years. They, like all living things, did a lot of adapting to a continually changing environment over those years. That in itself is a wonder.

Today, modern man no longer supposes, as the people of the Germanic North once did, that trees are the homes of spirits and gods. Today, he knows what they're made of and how they go about growing. But man has not lost that feeling of awe — perhaps a legacy of his early ancestry — that wells inside when he

lays eyes on those behemoths of the plant world.

Today, new developments in plant sciences have enabled man to create variations that nature may not have intended. We have many varieties of dwarf and compact trees that didn't exist even a decade ago. These new types, together with our increased knowledge of a tree's adaptability and growing requirements, enable us to enjoy the beauty and majesty of many trees — without their enormity — inside our homes as well as out. Many of our favorite trees can be grown in pots right in our own living rooms. These indoor trees are not examples of the largest plants on Earth, but they are examples of the largest ones in our indoor environment. As such, they act as eye-catching, often breath-taking focuses of attention. And much, much more.

Man no longer has to brave the elements to curl up with a good book and a glass of wine beneath the boughs of a spreading chestnut tree. He can enjoy those same aesthetic pleasures right in his own living room.

In this book, I've chosen to include some tree-sized plants, shrubs, and vines that are not by definition trees. Many of these because of their size make exciting additions to any decorating scheme. It would be a shame to omit them because they do not comply technically with the focus of this book. Such plants as the Oregon grape (*Mahonia aquifolium*) and mock orange (*Philadelphus coronarius*) are both shrubs. The jade plant (*Crassula argentea*) reaches a treelike height of 10 feet in the wild but is actually a slow-growing succulent indoors. The familiar pineapple (*Ananas comosus*) is a slow-growing bromeliad, while the banana tree (*Musa ensete*) is actually an herb. But all these plants make interesting tree-sized additions and are easy to grow in nearly any home or office.

A few words about flowering: Some trees and shrubs flower quite easily under average indoor growing conditions (camellias, for instance) while others do so only reluctantly. Many plants require optimum conditions, such as those available to them in their natural habitat or in a carefully tended greenhouse, to produce blooms. All plants, of course, must be mature before they flower (flowering is actually a plant's means of sexually reproducing itself).

Except in those cases where flowering trees are not known to flower indoors, I describe the bloom in the listing at the end of this book. The fact that I describe the flowers means the tree is known to have grown and flowered in somebody's house, although conditions and requirements may prevent it from doing so in yours. But indoor plants shouldn't be selected on the basis of their blooms. They should be chosen for their overall personalities: what they add to your home's décor as well as to your sense of personal enjoyment. Then, if it flowers (or if you can adjust your home's conditions to induce it to flower), it's a little like winning your local lottery. You've gained an unexpected bonus for your trouble, a reward for your patience and your sensitivity to some of the most amazing and beautiful creations on Earth.

How to Choose

Many considerations go into selecting a tree or a tree-sized shrub for your home. If you buy a tree, you'll probably spend between $5 and $75 or more, depending on the type, size, and availability of tree and where you buy it. If you harvest the tree yourself by digging it up and transplanting it, it'll still cost you in time and effort as well as the tender loving care necessary to nurture it from a small sapling to a mature specimen. If you hastily select the wrong tree or shrub, you come out on the short side of the investment.

On the other hand, with a little forethought and planning, a bit of investigative research and dreaming, your new acquisition can quickly become one of the most valuable possessions in your home. It's hard to understand, but when you round out your decorating pattern with a beautiful maple, elm, birch, or *zelkova* (a tree whose attractive lines and elegant features never disappoint), you grow closer and more attached to that living, growing organism with each passing day. And there's not a time when you walk past it while going about your business that you don't pause to admire it.

Furthermore, when you actually plan a tree into your home's surroundings, you increase the pleasure of ownership even more through anticipation. Let's consider a few examples.

- You have a home with a small dinette area where the family gathers for breakfast and lunch. On one wall is a giant picture window or, better yet, sliding glass doors leading to the patio or deck. You position an arching, graceful *Dracaena* next to the glass. In its pot, you arrange a colorful splash of long-blooming pansies around the tree's trunk. From spring through fall, the tree's small bright-green leaves add excitement and a touch of the outdoors to your meals. In winter, the pansies are a work of art set against a backdrop of frosty, silvery panes.
- Your family room is decorated modestly with wicker furniture and bamboo wall hangings. In one corner hangs a wicker swing lined with soft, colorful pillows. Above the swing unfold the long fanlike leaves of a banana tree, complete with fruit bunches. You can almost hear Harry Belafonte.
- Your teenage daughter's bedroom is a combination of styles best described as modish-messy. In one corner sits a stylish desk (about $395) with matching swivel chair and a fluorescent desk lamp for doing homework. In an opposite corner rests a $15 fig alongside several $3 throw pillows, and your daughter (of course), busy texting her friends instead of doing her homework.

So, it's easy to envision trees and shrubs being part of nearly any area of your home. As long as it gets enough food, water, and light, it's literally home free.

Speaking of Light

At one time, indoor gardening was restricted to the amount of natural light entering the house through the windows. That severely limited the number of plants you could grow and where you could grow them. Not so today. With a wide array of plant lights, soil and planting media, fertilizer, decorator pots, and assorted paraphernalia available, you can pretty much rest assured that, if you see a place just begging for a plant, you can make it happen. But how do you decide what areas of your home or office are crying out, Plant me, plant me! That's something you'll be better prepared to answer after you have a basic understanding of what trees and shrubs can do for you. And vice versa. Here's just a sampling.

Trees add beauty. Perhaps the most fundamental reason for acquiring an indoor tree or shrub is to beautify a room. If you have a corner that definitely needs perking up — but you don't have $400,000 for a small Rembrandt or a Rubens — consider a tree or shrub. The last chapter of this book, Recommended Trees and Shrubs, will help you in your selection. It lists various plant details and sizes. It contrasts large-leaved and small-leaved trees, flowering and nonflowering trees, trees that require bright light and those that thrive in shade, stately and casual trees. Decide on what tree or shrub you'd like to see growing in that empty corner, and then check out how much money (if any) you'll have to spend to put it there. The results? Instant beautification.

Trees add serenity. If you have a study or a hobby area that needs a little extra touch to set it apart from the more mundane rooms in your home, consider a tree. An evergreen might be best (not all evergreen trees are conifers or junipers; some are exotic-looking, and others are hard to distinguish from the deciduous leaf-shedding varieties so familiar outdoors). One

advantage to an evergreen is that its needles or leaves will generate their calming effect all year round. Without that fall raking!

Trees add drama. If you have a foyer or another drab area of the house that could use a centerpiece to impress and delight visitors entering your home, consider a massive, dramatic, easy-to-grow tree, either evergreen or deciduous.

Trees add warmth. If your home suffers from "colditis" — that hard-to-explain but always depressing feeling of impersonality in so many homes — add a grouping of small or medium-sized trees and shrubs.

Together with some companion plants (see Chapter 13), they're sure to add warmth and personality to your surroundings.

One Man's Meat

In the meantime, remember that no one's ideal is the same as the next one's. The first time I visited the home of one of my good friends — a doctor at Methodist Hospital in Madison, Wisconsin — I was impressed with a large palm and a hanging asparagus fern. There were two or three other small houseplants in the home. "They're nice," my friend confided that evening, "but I almost think we have too many plants in here."

A couple of weeks later, my doctor friend and his wife returned the visit. They raved about the warm, homey feeling of my place, which was much smaller than their mini-manse. I had a dozen trees, shrubs, and tons of small houseplants scattered throughout the house.

My point is this: don't arbitrarily assume your home is saturated with plants. I've often thought the most ideally decorated home would be one that was stocked first with plants, fountains, and rock gardens and rounded out afterward with furniture. That might be a little extreme for the average person to cope with. And, I admit, it might be a bit impractical. But in nearly a dozen years of indoor gardening, I've yet to find a home with too many plants in it.

Of course, when you plan the addition of a tree or shrub, take into consideration the predominant style of your furniture. Whether your rooms are Louis XIV, Victorian, Spanish, or Danish modern, what you add to them makes a difference. If you plan on adding greenery to a room that's primarily Oriental in design, you'll be wise to pass up the urge to acquire a *Dracaena marginata*, a rubber plant (*Ficus elastica*), or a golden locust (*Robinia friesia*). The general shape and color of these trees' foliage would detract from, rather than add to, your Oriental motif. Instead, consider the elliptical-leaved weeping fig

(*Ficus benjamina*) or one of several yews, Japanese maples, or aralias.

On the other hand, if your decor is traditional Spanish filled with dense, dark wood, you'd be better off considering some of the larger-leaved, more dramatic trees such as the ubiquitous rubber plant (*Ficus elastica*), the *Dracaena fragrans*, or the fiddle-leaf fig (*Ficus lyrata*).

Unlocking the door to successful decorating with houseplants is no simple matter. Many considerations are involved if you want to do it right. Not the least of these concerns is managing to balance your own predilections with the aesthetic beauty of specific trees or shrubs adding to your home's decor. While my living room is primarily classic American, my study is predominantly Early American clutter. It's a combination of eras — some modern along with Early American, plus a little Philippine wicker and "office functionality."

In my living room, I've selected plants that complement the decor. I use thick-leaved trees, full shrubs, and ferns to add warmth. A leathery-leaved lemon tree and an ornate fig look perfectly at ease alongside a thick, bushy rubber plant.

For my study, I've selected trees and shrubs mostly for their aesthetic beauty and air-cleansing abilities rather than for their ties to the decor. The result is a higher latitude of trees and shrubs than in my living room, with no particular loss in decorating value. My study enjoys a wide variety of greenery in the form of several black pine, apple, and orange trees, as well as in the delicate curvature of a weeping fig.

Other Considerations

One of the primary choices you'll face when decorating with trees is the overall size of the plant when mature. All plants can be headed back to control their height and pruned to limit their girth (more about how to do that later), but some species are more aggressive growers than others. To keep them in check, you might end up reaching for the pruning shears four or five times a year to prevent them from growing out the windows. How much wiser had you selected a species that grows no larger than your room can accommodate, or at least a slow grower that requires only occasional pruning.

Conversely, it wouldn't make sense to place a 6-foot Chinese rose tree (*Prunus triloba*) in a room that boasts a soaring 20-foot ceiling. The rose tree would make a better candidate for a family room of more modest proportions, while neem or *Ficus* trees would be better accommodated in a setting where space is as unlimited as the plants' growth habits themselves.

Ideally, a tree destined to become the focal point of any room should be maintained at about three-fourths the room's height once fully grown. A tree of that height dominates the space without seeming to crowd it. Other trees and shrubs ranging from shortest to tallest serve to round out the appearance of the room and provide continuity to the eye and a warm, comfortable feeling for the soul.

Remember the Tree's Palette

As a rule, several different characteristics of trees combine to create what many horticulturists call their *palette*. These components include size, form (at maturity), texture, bark, blossoms (maybe yes, maybe no), and fruit, if any. Also, since you may need to control a plant's height, we might add one other characteristic: growth rate.

Size when mature. In general, a tree's size when mature can be classified in one of three categories in the wild: small (under 20 feet), medium (under 40 feet), or large (40 feet and over). Most trees and shrubs can be grown indoors given the proper conditions (which include adequate light, humidity, nourishment, water, and container size or root space). Still, I've omitted some from general consideration in this book because their growth is too vigorous. They grow too tall too fast to be controlled even by the strictest pruning program. This group includes many of the tallest towering trees. Better candidates for indoor adaptation are medium- and short-growing trees and shrubs.

Form when mature. Trees, like people, come in many different shapes. Generally, they fit into one of five different categories:

- Columnar: very narrow with a rounded top (sentry maple)
- Fastigiate: narrow with a pointed top (Lombardy poplar)
- Pyramidal: conical (Douglas fir) with a rounded top
- Spreading: flattened (sugar maple) and broad or with an open headed airy top (silk tree)
- Weeping: drooping with pendulous branches (weeping willow, cherry, or magnolia)

Texture. This characteristic refers to the smoothness or roughness of the leaves, branches, and trunks of both evergreen and deciduous trees. It can be light — with delicate, feathery leaves (tree of heaven) and smooth trunks; medium — with more massive limbs and larger leaves (elm); or coarse — with heavy, chunky, leathery leaves (*catalpa*) and trunk.

Bark. This is an especially desirable characteristic in deciduous trees that shed their leaves for several months out of the year. If you decide on a deciduous tree, you may want to choose one with distinctive bark for year-round appeal, bark that flakes or peels or is especially colorful or deeply gnarled, for instance.

Blossom. We'll see later in the book which trees blossom under favorable conditions and which don't. In selecting flowering trees, you should take into consideration both the color and the size of the blossoms as well as the plant's period of bloom.

Fruit. In selecting a fruiting tree, you should consider the fruit's color and size as well as its function: is the fruit decorative, significant, or consumable? If not, why concern yourself?

Growth rate. I've avoided discussing in this book trees that grow too large too fast. But some trees that have a fast initial growth rate slow down when nearing their normal height at maturity. A number of these make excellent indoor specimens. They can be classified by the speed at which they grow.

- Slow: less than 1 foot a year (European birch or Norfolk Island pine).
- Medium: 1 to 2 feet a year (maple or cherry).
- Fast: 2 or more feet a year (poplar and some pine).

The growth rate is especially critical in trees intended for the house. It's somewhat less than wise to buy a 2-foot European birch sapling and wait a decade before seeing it reach the 20-foot height you were hoping for in its intended cathedral-like surroundings. And wouldn't it be a little counterproductive to bring a 5-foot poplar into a 7-foot room! As in all areas of life, a little planning and know-how can prevent a lot of disappointment in selecting a tree for your home. Understand your indoor tree's palette before bringing it into the house, and the only surprises you'll receive will be pleasant ones.

Remember the Tree's Requirements

There are only two sets of needs to consider when choosing a tree or shrub for your home: yours and the tree's. Of the two, the tree's are more important. While your needs can be modified to give you acceptable or even ideal results, the tree's demands aren't as flexible. If you don't give it what it needs for life and growth, it dies. Very much like a newborn child or a small puppy, an indoor tree is entirely dependent upon its "parents" for survival. More information on meeting a tree's indoor requirements appears later in this book.

Science Says

If your objective for planting trees and shrubs indoors is geared more toward creating a healthful environment than an aesthetically pleasing one, you can relax while you enjoy both. Plant your home for health, and the added aesthetics are sure to increase its market value. Plant for aesthetics, and your overall health will take a turn for the better.

Several conclusive scientific studies have recently proven that aesthetically appealing plantings — unusually large trees and shrubs — calm people down, lower their heart rate, make them more attentive, provide an enhanced learning environment, and lead to an increased sense of peace and relaxation.

Other studies have confirmed that planting indoor trees and shrubs for health reduces airborne contaminants, irritants, and bacterial/viral cells — a process known as *phytoremediation*. Trees and shrubs also absorb volatile organic compounds (VOCs) along with deadly carbon dioxide, which it converts into life-sustaining oxygen that the plants surrender back into their environment through respiration.

What else do trees and shrubs do? Unlike African violets and spider plants, which are great aesthetically, trees and shrubs have long been used to reduce noise from busy roadsides. More recently, research has shown another benefit:

interior plants can help reduce background noise in our homes and offices, too.

Our own studies indicate that plants and their leaves absorb, diffract, and reflect background noise, making the environment more comfortable for its occupants.

In one study, Peter Costa, a postgraduate student at South Bank University, London, found that some plants are particularly good at absorbing high sound frequencies. They are most dramatically effective in spaces defined as "acoustically live," places lined with hard surfaces such as tile, laminates, and hardwood floors.

Plants for beauty, emotional well-being, sound mitigation, and mental and physical health: It's a win-win situation for everyone.

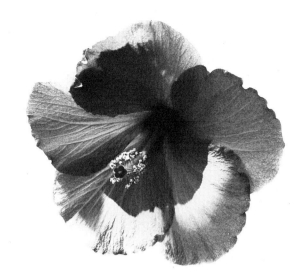

Chapter Two:

Greening Up for Health

WE LIVE IN A REMARKABLE TIME. And a remarkably frightening one. In our world, health, well-being, and occasionally even our very lives are threatened each and every day. And among the most significant, most harmful threats still on our radar: pollution.

Air pollution is high on the list of the most potent threats to people's health and well-being. Studies point out a direct link between urban air pollution — especially particulate pollution created by combustion-powered vehicles and power generation plants — and cardiovascular and pulmonary diseases. Long-term exposure to particulates, those tiny airborne particles smaller than 10 microns across (a human hair, by comparison, is 70 microns wide), has been shown to increase human illness and death rates from lung cancer, chronic obstructive pulmonary disease (COPD), and emphysema.

Exposure to other airborne pollutants, including sulfur dioxide (SO_2), nitrogen dioxide (NO_2), and ozone (O_3), also plays a role in developing diseases such as asthma, bronchitis, and various respiratory infectious diseases.[1]

Decades ago, European researchers investigating the risks of long-term exposure to traffic pollution discovered that people living near major roads (and therefore, one assumes, near exposure to lots of internal-combustion engines) were more likely to die from cardiopulmonary disease or lung cancer than their rural counterparts, merely because they were exposed to more harmful airborne particulates.

Medical researchers have also found a significant link between air pollution and cardiovascular health — heart disease! Reporting in the March 6, 2002, *Journal of the American Medical Association*, researchers examined long-term health data on half a million people to compare increases in air pollution levels with incidents of death. They discovered that when air pollution levels suddenly increase, so too do deaths from asthma, pneumonia, and emphysema. They also found an unexpected increase in the number of deaths related to heart attacks and stroke. Most surprising was the finding that when air pollution levels rise, so too do deaths from all causes, not only those related to the heart and lungs.

The reason is not that difficult to understand once you begin rooting around the science of human physiology. Air pollution causes oxidative stress that, in turn, triggers an inflammatory response in the lungs. That inflammation leads to the release of chemicals that impair heart function and blood pressure.

Several studies have found that exposure to high levels of air pollution stimulates bone marrow to release leukocytes and platelets. These are the killers that accumulate in pulmonary capillaries and so often result in heart attack or stroke.[2] So, the real enemy may not be so much the bad eating habits we've been warned about for decades, but pollution!

Corroborating those findings, the American Heart Association points out that someone dies from cardiovascular disease every forty seconds in the United States alone. Almost half of Americans have at least one of three main risk factors for heart disease: high blood pressure, high cholesterol, and smoking. Doctors tell their patients to exercise more, watch what they eat, and kick the cigarette habit to lower their cardiovascular risk — but there are other factors we must also recognize as impacting our heart health, such as air pollution exposure.

The Environmental Protection Agency conducts research and funds studies to advance our understanding of the link between air pollution and heart health. These research efforts support the National Ambient Air Quality Standards (NAAQS) and help provide better air quality for everyone. Most recently, researchers funded by EPA's STAR grant program at the University of Washington completed the Multi-Ethnic Study of Atherosclerosis Air Pollution Study (MESA Air), a decade-long analysis that revealed a direct link between air pollution and atherosclerosis, or a buildup of plaque in the coronary artery that can affect heart health.

Nearly one hundred percent of peer-reviewed articles summarizing the findings of MESA Air have been published since the research began in 2004, but in May 2016, *The Lancet* published a seminal article by lead investigator Dr. Joel Kaufman. It found that long-term exposure to particulate matter and nitrogen oxides at levels close to the NAAQS can prematurely age blood vessels and contribute to a more rapid buildup of calcium in the coronary artery. This calcium can restrict blood flow to the heart and other major blood vessels, increasing the likelihood of cardiovascular events such as heart attack and stroke.

While previous studies have linked air pollution and heart disease, this one provides "a finer degree of evidence that air pollution accelerates the process of atherosclerosis," according to Kaufman, thanks to the study's extensive length, diversity in subject participants, definitive scope, and rigorous system of data collection.[3]

Diabetics and Elderly at Risk

That's not the only bad news linking air pollution to cardiovascular disease. The medical journal *Epidemiology* examined Medicare records and hospital admissions in several U.S. cities and learned that, between 1988 and 1994, people suffering from diabetes were twice as likely as others to be admitted to a hospital with cardiovascular problems caused by airborne particulate pollution. They found, too, that persons seventy-five and older face a higher risk of cardiovascular injury than persons who have not been exposed to particulate pollution. Children are even more susceptible than adults. This is serious stuff.

As sobering as all of this is, it may not be the worst news about the effects of air pollution on human beings. Several Canadian studies conducted over the years concluded that animals exposed to the polluted air generated by a nearby steel mill actually suffered genetic damage, producing fewer offspring than their unexposed counterparts. Their damaged DNA was passed on to offspring by their fathers, although that fact does not mean that females are not also susceptible. The obvious implication is that steelworkers, who are mostly male, may be at extra risk of incurring similar DNA damage unless steps are taken to prevent exposure.

In a related study, researchers raised two groups of mice, the first half a mile downwind of a Lake Ontario steel mill and the second half twenty miles away. The mice housed closest to the polluted air source had twice as many mutations in their DNA as the mice breathing fresh air. The researchers concluded: "Our findings suggest that there is an urgent need to investigate the genetic consequences associated with exposure to chemical pollution through the inhalation of urban and industrial air."[4]

Protecting Your Lungs

While government, businesses, and environmental interests argue over the advantages of various economic, legislative, and technological solutions for cleaning up our polluted air, the vital issue facing individuals is how best to protect their own health today. Currently, over 75 million United States residents live in counties where the concentration of particulate matter smaller than 2.5 microns (PM2.5) exceeds safe levels.[5]

While living away from polluted cities may seem the obvious choice, that option is not available to everyone, nor is it always effective. Air currents and weather patterns can shift contaminated air from urban manufacturing centers into rural areas where pollution may accumulate in dangerous concentrations. Beyond that, modern farming practices rely upon mechanization, and mechanization means combustion engines that produce pollution in the form of particulates. So, too, do wood fires (a high source of airborne particulate), deteriorating automobile tires, agricultural chemicals, paint fumes (all those farmhouses have to be kept pristine!), and thousands of other rural particulate generators.

Staying indoors is no guarantee of experiencing better air quality, either. As numerous studies have recently shown, much of our exposure to fine particulates occurs inside the home! With no western breezes to move polluted air out of the house and the sealed "box" that can hold only a fixed amount of clean air,

accumulating particulates from deteriorating carpeting, padding, and wall surfaces alone, can pose a significant threat.

To make matters worse, many people at increased risk of health complications following exposure to high particulate concentrations, particularly the elderly and those suffering from cardiovascular and pulmonary diseases, spend as much as nine-tenths of their time indoors, raising still more concerns about the effects on health of a particulate-rich environment.

Air: The Great Equalizer

As indoor air pollution has grown in scope, so too have the number of people seeking air purifiers for relief from the problem. Home air-filtration products come in a wide range of types, all professing to do the same thing — cleanse the air. These products utilize electrostatic, UV radiation, water, and HEPA filtration technologies. Taking filtration one step further, a number of newer consumer products rely on ion-generating technology to eliminate indoor airborne pollutants, allergens, and viruses. They work by generating a flow of negative ions that charge and bind airborne particulate matter, which then clumps together to precipitate from the air.

Ion-generating devices have been shown to be effective against dust, cigarette smoke, pet dander, pollen, mold spores, viruses, and bacteria. In addition to eliminating harmful particulates from the air, negative ions also have a number of other unique health benefits.

Positively Negative Ions!

Just as positive ions build up in the atmosphere before a storm moves in, negative ions accumulate once the front passes. The surplus of negative ions has long been associated with improvements in mood and physical health. Research conducted in the last decade supports the view that negative ions have an overall positive effect on health.

One illuminating study in Germany involved isolating mice and rats in airtight sealed acrylic cases. The researchers filtered the ambient air to remove all negative ions from the cases. After being deprived of negative ions for some time, the death rate for the animals ballooned. Autopsies "strongly suggest that animal death is related to disturbances in neurohormonal regulation and pituitary insufficiency," according to the conclusion of the study.[6]

Other researchers at the Russian Academy of Sciences in Moscow discovered that negative ions are able to help protect the body from induced physical stress. When the researchers immobilized rats and exposed them to negative charges, they found that the ions prevented the development of pathological changes characteristic of the acute stress observed in the untreated rats. The only difference between the two groups was the protective action of negative ions.[7]

Taking the studies to a higher plane, British researchers exposed male subjects to negative ions and recorded their physiological responses, which included body temperature, heart rate, and respiration, both at rest and during exercise. The results showed that negative ions significantly improved all physiological states, especially during times of rest. The researchers concluded that negative ions are "biologically active and that they do affect the body's circadian rhythmicity."[8]

Yet another study, at the Institute of Theoretical and Experimental Biophysics of the Russian Academy of Sciences in Pushchino, Russia, found that subjects exposed to negative ions experienced increased levels of the protective antioxidant enzyme, superoxide dismutase. The researchers also discovered minute amounts of H_2O_2 and concluded, "The primary physiochemical mechanism of beneficial biological action of negative air ions is suggested to be related to the stimulation of superoxide dismutase activity by micromolar concentrations of H_2O_2 (hydrogen peroxide)."[9]

What It All Means

In short, negative ions with all of the biochemical reactions they produce are good for people and positive for the environment while virtually just the opposite is true of positive ionization.

While there has been growing signs of promise in the continuing battle against air pollution, especially in the emissions of lead, sulfur dioxide (SO_2), nitrogen dioxide (NO_2), and ozone (O_3), air pollution in the form of particulates, or microscopic airborne solid particles, remains a troubling health problem. In addition to damaging the lungs and heart, particulate pollution, according to medical researchers, is especially harmful to children, the elderly, and some sensitive populations, such as those afflicted with diabetes, cardiopulmonary disease, and other maladies.

Trees and shrubs — and, in fact, all plants in general — help to generate negative ions, both indoors and out. The critical concern, though, is for improved human health where we spend most of our time — indoors. And the good news is that trees and shrubs can do an exceptionally efficient job of cleaning up the indoor air we breathe.

The Orlando-based blog, *Pros Who Know*, links data it pulls from NASA research that examines the best, most effective means of generating purer air for use in shuttles, stations, and other areas where space is confined and air exchange is minimal. In doing so, the Agency identified the Big Three of plants best suited for cleaning the air: *Areca* palm, mother-in-law's tongue, and money plant. Subsequent studies have turned up some other top contenders for the title, including English ivy, *Ficus*, peace lilies, and *Gerbera* (Gerber) daisies, all of which have the added benefit of looking attractive.

Adding trees and shrubs to your indoor environment has other benefits, as well. In addition to neutralizing carbon dioxide and harmful chemicals and generating life-sustaining oxygen, plants improve indoor air quality in several ways.

Helping to maintain humidity levels. Dry indoor air is the cause of a host of respiratory problems, particularly during the winter when most houses and work environments are completely shut in. Plants help combat dry air by emitting water vapor during the process of transpiration — some more than others.

A recent study of seven common houseplant taxa or groups representing a variety of leaf types and sizes, measured the ability of various plants to absorb carbon dioxide and contribute relative humidity under a wide range of indoor light levels. Of the plants studied, two — various cultivars of *Spathiphyllum wallisii* (peace lily) and *Hedera helix* (ivy) — proved most efficient at accomplishing the task at hand.[10]

The takeaway from the study? If you want a quick pick-me-up for your home or work environment, load up on these plants. As a bonus, both make attractive companion plants for your larger trees and shrubs!

Producing negative ions. Plant leaves also generate negative ions, similar to many air purifying machines. Negative ions attach themselves to particles such as dust, mold spores, bacteria, and allergens, effectively removing them from the air we breathe and keeping them out of our bodies. The presence of negative ions is credited for boosting psychological health, productivity, and well-being.

The negative ions that indoor plants generate, while minimal in the overall scope of outdoor air pollution and airborne particulates, help to establish a microclimate indoors second to none. Outdoors, trees, shrubs, and other plants act as air cleansers/purifiers to clean up the air in our neighborhoods, towns, cities, and wherever else plants are being grown. A healthy outdoor microclimate, especially when combined with a healthy indoor environment, is the best means we have of combating the health hazards of air pollution on an individual basis.

The negative impact on health from ignoring the effects of air pollution in our environment is perhaps nowhere more evident than in the relatively small, picturesque town of Trinidad, Colorado. Set in the southwestern corner of the state, it butts up to northern New Mexico and Trinidad's sister hamlet of Raton. Sitting squarely inside a bowl whose lip rises to the south and west of the town while flattening out to the north and east, Trinidad was for decades home to the miners who worked in the coal pits of the Raton Basin south and west of town. The mines are mostly deserted now, but since the 1980s, companies have been drilling new gas wells to extract coalbed methane from the remaining coal seams. All those years of mining operations in the pre-EPA days of blissful ignorance spewed numerous sources of particulate, harmful gases, and chemicals into the air. Eventually, they made their way into the watershed, and both air and water pollution wended their way down the hillsides and into the front yards, homes, and offices of the town.

As a result, Trinidad's physicians, who number far below the national average by population, have been working overtime treating a community with growing incidents of cardiovascular disease, diabetes, and pulmonary disease. The overall air quality in Trinidad is ranked 85 on a scale of 100 (the higher, the better), based upon the EPA's newly revised measurement of hazardous air pollutants, the National Air Toxics Assessment.[11] This analysis provides models of respiratory illness and cancer risks down to the zip-code level. It produces much more accurate detail and insight into air pollution than had been available in previous analyses based solely upon results from air-monitoring stations placed sporadically around the region.

Water quality in Trinidad is also lacking, not unusual where there is a higher incidence of air pollution and airborne particulates than usual. On a scale of 100, Trinidad ranks 77 (again, the higher, the better). Note that this figure is a measure of watershed quality and not the quality of the water that comes out of the residents' faucets. Still, as the EPA is quick to note, a healthy watershed is closely related to high-quality drinking water. The EPA has a sophisticated method of measuring watershed quality using fifteen indicators such as pH, chemicals, heavy metals, and bacteria.

For the residents of Trinidad, all these indicators translate into an 85.7 percent risk of getting cancer as opposed to a 59.9 percent risk statewide and 54.4 nationally. Similarly, the risk of developing respiratory disease is 83.3 percent in Trinidad compared to 64.3 statewide and 62.5 percent nationally.[12] Clearly, the correlation

between airborne pollutants, particulates, polluted watersheds, and overall health is very real — and, for Trinidad residents, very alarming.

But the verdict is in, and the science is real. Now, it's time for people to begin recognizing the tremendous number of healthful benefits to be derived from growing both indoor and outdoor plants and to start incorporating trees and shrubs into individual dwellings as well as throughout their communities at large. We need to demand more of our public officials and designers, architects, and contractors to provide for increased and improved growing spaces for trees and shrubs indoors — both in our homes as well as our commercial structures.

Would a house with at least one tree or shrub in every room be too much to ask? Hardly. The growing body of evidence correlating plants with human health is overwhelming. The ongoing challenge to human development over the next generation and beyond is how to achieve such as goal. We need to inform our city planners, contractors, and politicians of the healthful and curative benefits of indoor trees and shrubs and the negative ionization they produce to help awaken people to the illuminating benefits that only such greenery can provide.

Plants provide an incredible and marvelous environment of healthful living for everyone who embraces them, a horrifying and torturous environment of sickness, debilitating disease, and death for those who don't. People can't survive for long by breathing polluted air and drinking poisoned water.

So, whether you live in the high deserts of Utah and Arizona or in the mountains of the Canadian north; whether you call home a small rental apartment or a sprawling, rambling estate, we can all benefit from the beneficial, healing effects of trees and shrubs indoors.

And it's just about time that we did so.

Science Says

While many countries continue to make progress in the ongoing fight against air pollution, growing populations and the emissions they create remain a problem. Among the most persistent sources of dangerous pollutants are lead, sulfur dioxide (SO_2), nitrogen dioxide (NO_2), and ozone (O_3). Air pollution from particulates is a crucial health issue, especially indoors. In addition to damaging the lungs and heart, air pollution is recognized as being especially harmful to children, the elderly, and sensitive populations, including those suffering from diabetes, cardiopulmonary diseases, and other debilitating conditions.

To help battle indoor pollutants, a growing number of people are investing in costly and complicated air-filtration systems that generate negative ions to charge and precipitate airborne particulate matter for more efficient removal.

Negative ion-generating devices help to eliminate airborne pollutants, dust, cigarette smoke, pet dander, pollen, mold spores, viruses, and bacteria from the air. Research has shown that negative ions have a net positive effect on health, including improved mood, stabilized catecholamine regulation and circadian rhythm, enhanced recovery from physical exertion, and protection from positive-ion-related stress and exhaustion disorders. Research has also proven that plants grown indoors are among the most efficient and cost-effective means of generating negative ions and improving the quality of our indoor air. And that can lead to a healthier, happier life for everyone.

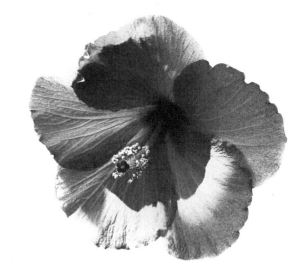

Chapter Three:

Greening Up for Home

NEARLY EVERYONE KNOWS that properly placed outdoor plants can help keep a house cooler in warm weather by basking it in shade. In fact, one young healthy tree can cool a building as effectively as ten room-sized air conditioners, according to one study conducted by the University of Vermont Extension.[1] Far fewer people know that indoor plants, particularly trees and shrubs, can also help reduce energy costs. The amount of money saved may not be as dramatic as with outdoor shade plants, but houseplants help reduce heating and cooling costs by adding humidity to the indoor environment.

Reduced Energy Costs

Plants release moisture into the air through the process of transpiration which takes place as moisture evaporates from the leaves. Paradoxically, this can both cool and warm a room, depending upon the ambient temperature. When plants release moisture into the air in a warm room, the result is a reduction in the temperature by as much as ten degrees, according to the University of Vermont Extension. On the other hand, according to a *U.S. News* article entitled "10 Ways to Save on Energy Costs This Winter," a cool but humid room feels warmer because the moist air holds heat better. That means in winter, you can set your thermostat a little lower than normal and still feel comfy![2]

But houseplants can help to save you money in other ways, too. Plants can reduce illnesses by as much as 23 percent by helping to eliminate harmful mold, bacteria, and toxins from the air. Through the process of photosynthesis, plants take in "bad" air and generate "good" air in the space surrounding the plant.

Bringing plants such as aloe, palms, herbs, and lilies into the house cleans the air of toxins—harmful pollutants released into the environment by everything from smoking to reading newspapers and handling other wood-pulp products. Growing plants indoors naturally filters out these contaminants, resulting in fewer trips to the doctor or hospital, less time lost from work, and greater overall savings.

But that's only one way plants can be a shot in the arm to your health. They can also strengthen the human immune system. The stronger your immune system is, the less susceptible you are to contracting potentially debilitating diseases such as cancer and Parkinson's disease. The more oxygen in the air, the stronger your immune system. The stronger your immune system, the better equipped your body will be to use that oxygen to fight off sickness and disease. And plants are the best natural oxygen generators known to man!

Depending upon the amount of ambient light available to your plants (or how many additional plant lights you bring into the room), consider growing potted palms in the parlor, Meyer lemon trees in the foyer, and tropical dwarf orange trees in the kitchen. Beyond their spectacular leathery greenery, citrus trees when in bloom will help sweeten the scent of any room naturally.

Psychology 101

But the benefits of houseplants don't stop there. Studies have shown that growing green plants indoors has great effects on stress levels as well. Think about how you feel less stressed whenever you go outside. The reason? All those fresh green plants surrounding you. The colors and scents do amazing things to perk us up mentally.

Lavender is a good example and an ideal plant for growing in well-lighted bedrooms to reduce stress and help you sleep at night. As a bonus, you can use it as a companion plant in a large pot containing an oxygen-generating tree or shrub. Bright flowering plants also help to fight off depression, making them the perfect addition for bedrooms.

And the benefits from growing indoor plants aren't limited to the four walls in which you find yourself. They can also contribute to better grades in school for the kids. That's because being surrounded by indoor plants helps calm children down so they can focus better on their studies.

Remember that all of us were, at one time long ago, conditioned to live out of doors where we could enjoy the beauty and health benefits of the plants surrounding us. By bringing some of that health-inducing nature inside with us, we provide ourselves with the ability to function better mentally as well as physically.

The numerous benefits of growing plants indoors go a long way toward explaining the booming popularity of indoor gardening today.

Less work: Gardening outdoors means lots of spade and hoe work while turning over the soil. It also means constant weeding to keep the invaders from sucking up valuable moisture and nutrients from the soil. And you have to stay constantly vigilant for harmful insects and diseases that often lurk just below the surface near your plants' vulnerable roots. Indoor gardening in sterilized soil eliminates all those problems and magnifies your chances for growing success.

Superior plants: In an outdoor world, your plants are pretty much at the mercy of Mother Nature. In an indoor system, you have complete control over nearly every aspect of your plant's growth — from lighting and moisture to soil nutrients and supplemental feedings. So, if you give your indoor plants what they need when they need it, you're virtually guaranteed success.

No time limits: Indoor gardening means you can grow plants all year long, not only during the peak outdoor growing season. Outdoor gardening means that, even during the peak growth months of summer, your plants are at the mercy of strong winds, hail, blazing sun, and torrential rains that can damage or even destroy them.

Fewer problems: While there's always a chance of running into some pesky pests indoors, gardening outdoors magnifies that chance a hundred-fold. The odds of a bug invading your home, finding a host plant to munch on, and propagating without your noticing the developing problem is miniscule. That means you spend less time chasing down pests while eliminating the need for harmful chemical pesticides, something difficult to do when tending to a large outdoor garden. Remember: Chemical pesticides aren't only an added expense but also an added source of toxins for you and your family to breathe in.

Create Instant Resale Value

If you own your home, a day will come when you're going to want to sell. Or even if you rent and want to sublet your apartment to someone else to finish out the lease, nothing short of a complete kitchen remodel can increase the perceived real value in your home or apartment more than a thoughtfully arranged, beautifully staged home filled with houseplants. Tall dramatic, textural trees and shrubs add a sense of elegance, stability, and openness to every décor, even to older smaller buildings. According to the Real Estate Associates of America, greenery in the home can make the difference between a sale and a walk-away.

"You can increase the value of your home by [providing] indoor plants," according to an article by G.I. Home Loans, a major lender and realtor specializing in residential property.

> Indoor plants can be a significant factor in staging a home. The welcome your home gives to visitors can make a good first impression … Healthy and attractive houseplants contribute to that WOW factor that can make the difference between a sale or not — or even between $300,000 and $250,000![3]

Research has shown that, when plants are present in a shopping area, people perceive the value of the merchandise being sold as greater compared to the same merchandise in an area without plants. "In one study," according to interior plantscape consultant Kathy Fediw, "consumers were willing to spend a conservative 12 percent more for products in an environment with trees (Wolf 2002)."[4] They also tended to shop longer and buy more in stores having plants, a statistic that has not gone unheeded in modern shopping malls and boutique shops.

Plants add a sense of luxury and prestige to a space, whether commercial, industrial, or residential. People particularly associate tropical plants with success and are more likely to be confident and secure in well-planted environments.

"Ferns, palms, and flowering plants are especially effective in creating a luxurious ambiance," Fediw says. "These plants are often used in the finest hotels, restaurants, and high-end luxury homes. Most successful corporate headquarters and prestigious office buildings have indoor plants."[5]

Boosting the resale value of your home by five, ten, or even twenty thousand dollars or more is as simple as placing your indoor plants where they'll do the best; and that's an advantage outdoor gardeners simply don't enjoy.

Plant a tree in the ground, and that's where it stays. Plant one in a container, and it's there for as long as you want it to be — no more, no less. You can change plants with the seasons, move your containers from one room to another, reposition plants within a room, swap out their containers for new ones, stagger your plantings for a continuous show or harvest, set the plants outside in the summer and bring them in during the winter, arrange them in groups, and even combine multiple plants in a single container for dramatic effect.

You can change color schemes to match your home's furnishings, add texture and drama to your home's design palette, and create specific moods to meet your needs and desires, all with a degree of flexibility unknown to conventional outdoor gardeners. And you can do all that while saving a ton of money on professional decorator bills!

And that's one of the most attractive and cost-effective features of container gardening of all.

Still More Reasons

Of course, those aren't the only reasons to consider growing trees and shrubs and, in fact, all your favorite plants indoors. Doing so can save you money by keeping your family healthy and well. Even when those occasional accidents happen, you can be assured of having just the right antidote at hand — as near as your closest flowerpot! By mixing companion plants and herbs with your larger trees and shrubs, you can have a year-round supply of everything from aloe vera to lavender, along with numerous other medicinal plants. See more about that in "Companion Planting for Health" later in the book.

Which Trees and Shrubs?

That brings up the inevitable question: Which trees and shrubs are best for indoor growth? In effect, that depends upon your environment. For starters, consider these variables.

Room height: How high are your ceilings? Whether they're 8-feet or 40-feet high will make a difference in how tall a specimen you should choose to grow. You can always check the height of all but the most aggressive tree or shrub even in an 8-foot-tall room by keeping the plant headed back — that is, pruning its top to control the plant's height; but that could quickly become tiresome. It's better to select a specimen whose growth is more suited to the room's height. We'll discuss the issue of short-, medium-, and tall-growing trees and shrubs later in the book.

Room lighting: Similarly, you shouldn't try growing high-light plants (plants that must have a strong light source in order to grow and remain healthy) in a low-light area. Sure, you can always subsidize weak lighting with grow lamps and through the use of various light-intensifying methods, such as installing mirror tiles on your wall or painting your walls white or light gray to reflect more light toward your plants; but, again, why go through all that trouble if you don't have to?

Also, selecting tropical trees and shrubs that require a high level of humidity to thrive and prosper can be a daunting task. Sure, you can mist the plants several times a day, and you can place trays filled with pebbles and water beneath them so that the evaporating liquid rises to surround the plant in humidity (theoretically, at least, although it sounds more efficient than it is in practice). But even those two approaches get old in a hurry unless you have nothing else to do with your time than wandering around the house with a spray bottle in your hand. Not to mention the problem of who's going to take over for you when you duck out of town for a weekend in the city.

To avoid these humidity problems, choose only plants with average humidity requirements — which, thankfully, include all but the most exotic trees and shrubs.

Summing Up

In the end, you'll find the best, easiest, and most popular trees and shrubs for indoor growth are the semi-tropical evergreens, although an increasing number of European and native North American evergreens are slowly winning people over with their growth habit, interesting form, texture, and overall hardiness. You can choose from other specimens, too, such as many of our common deciduous trees and shrubs — the ones that keep their leaves during the summer's growing season and shed them in the fall. But unless you have

lots of time to run around the house vacuuming up fallen leaves (and sometimes seedpods, as well), I'd suggest you steer clear of those species, a few of which are listed in the chapter on Recommended Trees and Shrubs.

Here's a short list of some plants you'll want to consider for your home. These are the ones that should be first on your list simply because they're time tested and ready to grow, All are available locally and through the mail, and are relatively hardy with a manageable growth rate.

These include the semi-tropical *Ficus benjamina* (weeping fig), *Dracaena marginata* (Madagascar dragon tree), *Schefflera arboricola* or *S. Actinophylla* (green or variegated umbrella tree), *Ficus lyrata* (fiddle-leaf fig), *Araucaria heterophylla* (Norfolk Island pine), *Yucca elephantipes* (giant yucca), *Crussala ovata* (jade plant), *Pachira aquatica* (money tree), and *Monstera deliciosa* (split-leaf philodendron). Some American "natives" gaining in indoor horticultural popularity include any of the dwarf citrus trees (kumquat, orange, lemon, and lime), *Prunus caroliniana* (North Carolina cherry), and some species of *Cupressus spp* (cypress), *Cedrus* spp (cedar), *thuja* (arborvitae), yew, and juniper.

For a more complete list of indoor-suitable trees and shrubs, check out the chapter "Recommended Trees and Shrubs."

Science Says

If you've ever wondered why it feels so good to be outdoors on a bright, sunny day, you're not alone. Scientists, too, have been asking themselves that question for decades. Here's what they've come up with.

That feeling of bliss that washes over you when you get away from it all isn't all in your head — not by a long shot. Spending time in the great outdoors has been scientifically proven to reduce stress levels, increase mental clarity, and rejuvenate both mind and body. Bringing the outside in through indoor trees and shrubs can help do the same. Here's how.

Reducing stress: Multitasking, particularly with electronic devices, is a leading cause of stress. A University of California, Irvine, study found that people who had access to email and received a steady flow of messages throughout the day had higher heart rates than those who were cut off from electronic communication.[6] Sitting down in a room full of plants is the next best thing to taking a walk in the park.

Focusing: Leaving your devices behind and spending time in your indoor "garden" can be calming for more metaphysical reasons. A study by the University of Illinois Landscape and Human Health Laboratory found that a natural environment allowed people to leave the stressors of their everyday lives behind and concentrate on the purity of nature. By focusing you mind, you can relax your body.[7]

Recharging: The human brain at rest utilizes one-fifth of all the energy the body produces. Under stress of mental challenge, that increases by 5 to 10 percent. When people are in a daydreaming state — something more easily achieved in nature's serene environment — their brains settle into what scientists call the default mode network (DMN), a complex circuit of coordinated communication between parts of the brain. It's an essential element of the thought process that enables us to understand human behavior, develop an internal code of ethics, and help us realize our identities.

Reducing hormones: A recent Dutch study suggests that people in a natural environment who perform repetitive tasks such as watering and pruning their plants have the ability to fight stress better than through other leisure activities. One group of participants was asked to read indoors after completing a stressful task, while the other group was instructed to tend to their plants for 30 minutes. The gardeners reported better moods and registered lower levels of the stress hormone, cortisol, than did the readers.[8]

Lowering blood pressure: In polluted indoor environments, the body is forced to work harder to get the oxygen it needs to function, thus raising your heart rate and blood pressure. A well-planted environment combats these problems.

Calming down: Research shows that breathing techniques can dampen the production of stress hormones while training your body to relate to stressful situations. Rapid shallow breathing (i.e., when you're under stress) triggers your body's sympathetic nervous system, or your "fight or flight" response. Slow, deep breathing (i.e., when you're in a natural environment) stimulates the body's parasympathetic reaction, which calms you down. Stopping to smell the roses, puts the brakes on your body's natural stress response.

Increasing oxygen levels: Levels of oxygen in your brain are tied to levels of serotonin, the neurotransmitter that affects your mood, appetite, memory, social behavior, and other processes. Too much serotonin causes irritability and tension; too little results in depression. Breathing fresh oxygenated air helps regulate your levels of serotonin and promote happiness and well-being.

Boosting ion levels: The negative ion-rich oxygen found in a well-planted environment produces relaxation. Negatively ionized air, like that produced by large trees and shrubs, promotes alpha brain waves and increases brain wave amplitude, which creates an overall mind-clearing and calming effect.

Increasing serotonin levels: Nature's calming effect is produced not only in the air, but also in the soil. Research done by scientists at the University of Colorado at Boulder shows that *Mycobacterium vaccae*, a harmless bacteria commonly found in soil, can act as a natural antidepressant by increasing the release and metabolism of serotonin in parts of the brain that control cognitive function and mood. These bacteria can also decrease inflammation in your immune system, thereby squelching health problems ranging from heart disease to diabetes.[9]

So, if you want to live a healthier life indoors, you know what you need to do.

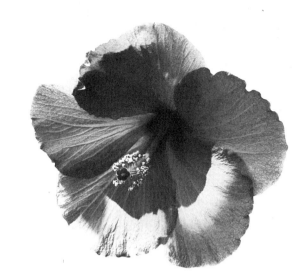

Chapter Four:

Greening Up for Work

RUNNING A BUSINESS can often prove demanding. Providing the right ambiance for your staff can play a critical role in your company's success. There are numerous ways to improve the ambiance of your business — some more obvious than others. Here are some of the elements you'll want to consider.

Increase employee morale: Maintaining a high morale among your employees is the most obvious way to increase productivity. A happy worker is a productive worker — that is, one who is content, focused, goal-driven, and results-oriented. That worker is more likely to produce more results more quickly and accurately.

Create an attractive workspace: People don't like to be in a work environment that's noisy, poorly lighted, and sparsely decorated. Such a setting grates on people's nerves and slows down their work output. On the other hand, people do like to be in an environment that provides them with a beautiful, comfortable, and peaceful setting. That type of setting generates increased work output and greater efficiency.

Construct a peaceful setting: Just as people dislike ugly surroundings, they hate a grating, noisy, distracting work environment. By stripping the workplace of elements that tend to generate tension and replacing them with items that create a calming effect, you'll find increased productivity and less turnover in your employee ranks.

Build a secure work environment: Nobody likes to work in an environment that puts them on edge where they have to worry about who's watching their every move (and why!). That's where constructing a secure cubbyhole type of environment can work wonders. Make your staff feel as if they're in their own protective cocoons, and you'll have happier, healthier employees.

Provide a healthy workplace: If your work environment is stuffy, dry, smelly, or otherwise less than desirable, take a tip from the experts and change all that around. An undesirable workplace creates dissatisfied employees who are more apt to get sick. And a sickly worker is not a productive employee; a healthy worker is.

What's the Cost?

If you find yourself asking what making all those changes for your employees' welfare and your company's bottom line will cost you, you're not alone. Neither are you in a minority if you assume such a cost to be in the thousands of dollars. But you'd be wrong. There is, in fact, a simple, quick, and cost-effective way to provide an attractive, peaceful, secure, and healthy work environment. In a word: plants.

Among the least expensive of makeovers available, adding plants to the environment can cost anywhere from a few to several hundred dollars. Depending upon its size, an office can be improved to provide a more genteel work

experience that, in turn, increases employee production, reduces turnover, slashes worker errors, and heightens employee satisfaction.

Hiring It Out

Of course, not everyone feels up to the task of buying plants, bringing them to the workplace, arranging them for greatest benefit, and maintaining them when there are other jobs to be done. If that's an issue in your business or workplace, you might consider using an interior landscaping company to shoulder the heavy lifting. An indoor plant specialist can take over the task of choosing the best types of plants to complement the environment.

One of the greatest benefits of using an interior landscaping company comes after the plants have arrived. Once they have been placed, it's assuring to know that someone is watching over them — watering them, providing adequate light for growth, and keeping an eye out for insects and other pests that could quickly decimate a plant.

Most leading specialists in indoor landscaping have personnel trained in plant maintenance. That's important because simply bringing a plant into the office and abandoning it is sure to spell disaster; and researchers have shown that plants in poor health have a detrimental effect on morale and productivity — not exactly the goal you were shooting for.

And not only do plants change the workplace for the better, they also add the appearance of changing the workplace for the good. A study by Engelbert Kötter in collaboration with the Bavarian State Ministry of Nourishment, Agriculture and Forestry found that healthy plants in offices actually enhanced employees' perception of the company's well-being by improving the "comfort factor" of the offices because people tend to react positively to plants and perceive the use of indoor plants as a sign of success.[1]

Humans Relate to Plants

Part of the reason workers react so positively to plants is that all human beings have an innate desire to be connected to nature, a concept that scientists call *biophilia*. Simply adding some greenery in the form of indoor plants can have major benefits for employees and the companies for which they work. Here are some specific reasons you should invest in plants for your place of employment.

Plants reduce stress: A 2010 study by the University of Technology of Sydney, Australia, showed significant reductions in stress among workers when plants were introduced to their workspace. Results included a 37% reduction in tension and

anxiety; a 58% drop in depression or dejection; a 44% decrease in anger and hostility; and a 38% reduction in fatigue.

Although the study's sample size was small, researchers concluded: "This study shows that just one plant per workspace can provide a very large lift to staff spirits, and so promote wellbeing and performance."[2]

Plants increase productivity: Employees' productivity jumped 15% when previously "lean" work environments were filled with a mere handful of houseplants, according to a 2014 research by the University of Exeter. Adding only one plant per square meter improved memory retention and helped employees score higher on other basic tests, according to researcher Dr. Chris Knight. "If you are working in an environment where there's something to get you psychologically engaged you are happier and you work better."[3]

Plants reduce sickness and absenteeism: The 2015 Human Spaces report, which studied 7,600 office workers in 16 countries, found that nearly two-thirds (58%) of workers had no live plants in their workspaces. Those whose environments incorporated natural elements reported a 15% higher well-being score and a 6% higher productivity score than those whose offices didn't include such elements.[4]

Some experts argue further that adding plants to the work environment can help to reduce the risk of "sick building syndrome," where people in a building suffer from symptoms of illness or feel unwell for no apparent reason, although evidence to back up these claims is not widely available.

A small study by the Agricultural University of Norway in the 1990s found that the introduction of plants to one office was linked to a 25% decrease in symptoms of ill health, including fatigue, concentration difficulties, dry skin, and even eye-and-nose irritation![5]

"The presence of plants can probably result in a positive change in the psychosocial working environment," said professor Tøve Fjeld in a 2011 blog post.

> The resultant feeling of well-being also affects how the individual assesses his/her state of health. Against the background of the psychobiological identity and mankind's positive reaction to nature we can assume that plants have a particular effect on the sense of well-being. This is evidenced by the fact that the occurrence of symptoms linked to the indoor atmosphere was reduced.[6]

Plants attract job applicants: Commenting on the 2015 Human Spaces report when it was released, organizational psychology professor Sir Cary Cooper said:

> The benefit of design inspired by nature, known as biophilic design, is accumulating evidence at a rapid pace. Looking at a snapshot of global working environments, up to one in five people have no natural elements within their workspace, and alarmingly nearly 50% of workers have no natural light. Yet a third of us say that workplace design would affect our decision to join a company. There's a big disparity here and one that hints at workplace design only recently rising to prominence as a crucial factor.[7]

Plants clean the air: While humans need oxygen to survive, plants absorb a gas we find poisonous — carbon dioxide — an element that plants combine with water and light to produce energy through photosynthesis.

In the 1980s, scientists at NASA discovered that plants were also adept at removing chemicals such as benzene, trichloroethylene, and formaldehyde from the air, making it cleaner for humans to breathe. More current research led by Fraser Torpy, director of the University of Technology's Plants and Indoor Environmental Quality Research Group in Sydney, has found that indoor plants can help reduce carbon dioxide levels by about 10% in air-conditioned offices and by some 25% in buildings without air conditioning.

Plants reduce noise levels: By actually absorbing sounds (as opposed to insulating against noise), plants help to reduce the distracting effects of background office chatter, clacking keyboards, and other noise pollutants. Positioning several larger potted plants along the periphery and in the corners of a room produces a measurable positive benefit, according to a 1995 paper by researchers at London South Bank University.[8]

Plants boost creativity: The 2015 Human Spaces report found that employees whose offices included natural elements scored 15% higher for creativity than those whose offices didn't. The reason is something known as Attention Restoration Theory, which suggests that looking at nature — and sometimes even *images* of nature — can shift the brain into a different processing mode, making employees feel more relaxed and better able to concentrate.[9]

What Types of Plants?

Okay, so plants and offices were made for one another, which brings up the question: what types of plants? Obviously, durability is a factor, since workplace plants are apt to receive less attentive care than in-home plants. And the ability to survive in the generally harsher conditions of the work environment will prove useful. As for size, that should be determined by the space available for the plants. But another variance between plants is even more important, and that's their light requirements. Let's take a closer look.

Plants have different needs for the amount of light required to grow and be healthy. The three major categories are low-light, moderate-light, and high-light varieties. The low-light group make excellent candidates for dark areas, such as corners and small rooms with tiny or even no windows, such as bathrooms.

Plants that belong in this low-light group include *Agloanema, Pothos,* peace lily, *Philodendron,* snake plant, and ZZ plant.

Plants in the moderate-light group include the Bamboo Palm, *Schefflera,* Red Princess, Kentia Palm, *Philo Xanadu,* and the Lady Palm.

Plants in the high-light group include the sago palm, Ming aralia, ponytail palm, fiddle-leaf fig, olive tree, and the yucca cane.

For a wider selection of plants suited for office use, check out the list of plants in the back of the book.

So, plants for the office or other work environment? Absolutely. They're more than just a pretty face. Plants can make the difference to a business between success and failure and between survival and demise. They can lower absenteeism and employee turnover and increase profits and worker satisfaction.

In short, if you're working in a plant-free environment, it's time you changed your outlook and took a positive step into a healthier, more productive future.

Science Says

Offices devoid of plants are "the most toxic space" into which a human being can be placed. That's what several psychologists said in a September 2014 study that claims workers perform better when household plants are added to workplaces. In other words, "green" is better than "lean."

Chris Knight from Exeter University in Devon, England, together with several fellow psychologists, have been studying the issue for more than a decade. They concluded that employees are 15% more productive when "lean" workplaces are filled with only a few houseplants. The reason? Employees who actively engage with their surroundings make better, more satisfied workers.[10]

Collaborating with academics from four universities in Australia, the UK, and the Netherlands, Knight had wondered for years why Spartan offices have been in vogue so long. "If you put an ant into a 'lean' jam jar, or a gorilla in a zoo into a 'lean' cage, they're miserable beasties," he said. People in "lean" offices are no different.

In the last 18 months, Knight and his colleagues have visited workplaces in a call center in the Netherlands and the offices of a large city auditor in London to show how the addition of some greenery could quickly improve performance.

The auditors had spent "a lot of money" on their office, according to Knight. "They had very expensive desks … banners that were just to do with the company … it was a beautifully sparse environment."[11] The call center was similarly stripped bare. Knight said some companies he knew of had even taken to fixing computer keyboards to desks and taping down staplers to ensure tidy lines of vision. But that failed to improve levels of worker performance. Only when Knight introduced plants into the offices at the rate of one for each square meter did employee performance on memory retention and other basic tests improve dramatically.

"What was important was that everybody could see a plant from their desk. If you are working in an environment where there's something to get you psychologically engaged, you are happier and you work better."[12]

Knight said he hopes the 18-month project will put to rest the practice of maintaining "lean" offices in lieu of plants once and for all.

Alex Haslam, from the University of Queensland's School of Psychology, who co-authored the study, added: "The 'lean' philosophy has been influential across a wide range of organizational domains. Our research questions this widespread conviction that less is more. Sometimes less is just less."[13]

As Knight had discovered, numerous studies have shown that the use of plants in the workplace has verifiable benefits when it comes to improving morale and productivity within the workforce. Indoor plants provide aesthetic value, improve air quality, and reduce stress while maximizing business profitability.

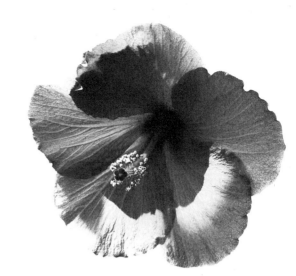

Chapter Five:

Bringing the Outdoors In

I DON'T FOLLOW any hard-and-fast rule about where I get my indoor trees and shrubs. Usually, after considering my home's suitability for growing a particular plant, I take two factors into account: availability and price. My Bohemian heritage comes into play when I find a tree I want online or in a plant shop, nursery, or mail-order catalog. The first question I ask myself is "How much?" and the second is "Can I find it cheaper somewhere else?" The cheapest trees around, of course, are free. And that's a very attractive price, indeed. We'll talk about hunting those down later. But for now, let's talk about where to buy certain trees that must be bought and how much to pay for them without feeling you've been had.

When I lived in a northern climate, I had to turn to a plant specialty shop for those tropical and subtropical trees (exotic trees) that people living in Florida,

Arizona, and California can often have for free. But I learned early in life never to bite on the first offering.

While researching an article on houseplants years ago, I fell in love with the delicate fronds and graceful, sweeping trunk of *Dracaena marginata*. The first one I ran across was in a large well-appointed plant shop in Chicago. The main trunk stood six feet tall and had three branches, each topped with lush green foliage. Gorgeous! The price? A lush green $100 — more than I was willing to spend at the time.

So I started shopping around. In each plant store and nursery, I checked out the size and price of the *Dracaenas* first thing. I found one with a single stalk and two branches for $60. In another shop, I found a pot with two separate stalks for $55. A third shop featured three stalks for $50 — and I was ready to buy. But before pulling out my wallet, I talked to the store's owner and griped a bit about how expensive the plant was. He hemmed and hawed before finally telling me that, if I cared to wait, the store would be featuring its annual clearance sale in a month — 50 percent off on all plants! The only problem was, there were no special orders. The sale was good only on plants already in the store. I decided to gamble and hope the *Dracaena marginata* would still be there one month later.

Well, I was the first customer through the door on sale day, and the *Dracaena* of my dreams was still there. I bought what had seemed at $50 to be the best-priced Drac in town for only $25. It's called shopping around, and considering that many plant shops carry a markup of from 60 to 200 percent and more, I recommend nothing less to anyone about to make a major plant purchase.

The plants you'll have to buy to display in your home collection depend upon where you live. Obviously, if something you want doesn't grow wild right outside your door — and you can't convince a friend or neighbor who has the same plant to give you some of its progeny — you'll have to either part with the money or settle on something else. Besides large tropical and subtropical trees, most people find they must buy their small ornamental shrubs and trees as well as dwarf

fruit trees and hybrids for their home collection — such as ornamental pear, ornamental crab, and dwarf apple.

Watch Out for Warning Signs!

Most plant shops and nurseries I've visited during my decades of indoor growing have had fairly good, strong, healthy stock and knowledgeable salespeople. I said most, not all. I've been to some shops and nurseries where one plant looked worse than the next and nobody on the payroll knew a banana tree from a marigold. That type of shop you can live without. Often, disreputable businesses like those continue to flourish because they're the only game in town. The management thrives on its customers' general ignorance about plants. But you don't have to be among the uninitiated.

When you walk into a plant shop or nursery, take the time to inspect the plants — all plants, including flowers, small houseplants, and cacti. Examine the leaves of plants in various locations within the shop. Are they healthy looking? Or are they puffy, swollen, and sagging? Are they green (or whatever color they're supposed to be), or are they brown and crinkly or yellow along the edges? Especially check the fleshy-leaved plants (*Ficus, Croton, Schefflera,* etc.). Turn the leaves over gently and look closely for signs of insects. Some bugs are no larger than the tiniest grain of pepper, so you have to take your time and inspect carefully. What you're doing, of course, is trying to determine whether or not the retailer buys its plants from a reputable wholesaler and whether or not they're disease- and insect-free.

Be especially watchful for ants crawling around the leaves of certain plants, particularly in outdoor nurseries, that may well mean an infestation of aphids. Aphids are tiny green, red, or white sucking insects that can draw the life out of many different species of plants. Ants often seek out the aphids, enslaving them for the honey-like secretions aphids expel. While ants do little or no harm to the plants themselves, their presence should serve as a warning sign.

And don't content yourself with disease- and insect-free plants. Check the main stems of several larger plants. Are there any scars where branches or leaves have recently fallen off? A few scars, of course, are normal — shedding is part of a plant's natural growth cycle. But an abnormally high number of wounds indicates something serious could be going on.

Also check out the pot size in relation to the plant size. Slipshod, make-a-quick-buck wholesalers couldn't care less about properly potted plants. They often ship greenery in the smallest pots possible to reduce their potting and shipping costs at your expense. Are the roots heaving out of the top of the pot or growing out of the drainage holes at the bottom? If so, steer

clear. The plant's root system could be seriously compromised.

If you find anything wrong with the store's plants, don't hesitate pointing it out to the manager. Often, you can gain a better insight into management integrity from watching a manager's reaction to your complaint than from inspecting a thousand plants yourself. If he shrugs his shoulders and has a take-it-or-leave-it attitude, skip it. He's in business for one reason and one reason only — to separate you from your money.

If, on the other hand, the manager appears genuinely concerned and takes steps to point out other similar but healthier plants from which you may choose — and possibly even reminds you of the store's guarantee that you can return failed plants within a reasonable period of time — you might give him a chance. If he's sincere, he cares more about his reputation and that of the store than about trying to rip you off. And that's the kind of place where you want to do business.

Free Trees

Now we come to one of my favorite methods of procuring trees: collecting. Luckily, no one has yet managed to place a patent on Mother Nature. That means the fruits of her labor belong equally to anyone interested in plucking. However, you can't pick just any tree you happen to fall in love with. Farmers, ranchers, homeowners, and even Uncle Sam have been known to take a dim view of people digging around on their property.

But there are plenty of rich hunting grounds elsewhere. On your own property, for example. Or in unpaved city alleyways. Or on public property not designated as a recreation area. (A state or national park or forest really frowns on plant removal!)

Often, seeds from neighborhood elms, maples, willows, or other favorites find their way right to your back door and, about the time the first robins return north, begin sprouting up and budding. These are the same shoots you may have treated as nuisance weeds in the past, chopping them down with the power mower on that first tedious pass in the spring. The same is true with evergreen cypress and arborvitae trees. Pay attention to what's growing right under your own feet.

Another excellent source of free trees is unincorporated land outside city or town limits. It may well be fair game for tree collectors (check with your county agricultural agent to be sure) … within the bounds of common sense, of course. For example, it's ecologically foolish and just plain ridiculous to take more trees or larger trees than you can successfully dig and transplant at home. And, when removing a tree from its natural habitat,

do it thoughtfully. Be sure to return the ground to its natural order; don't leave gaping holes for others to stumble into. And no cigarette butts or crinkled packs lying around, either, or damaged trees left standing near the ones you remove. Remember: None of us owns this planet; each of us is only a visitor.

What Time of Year?

When to go foraging for indoor trees is every bit as important as where you go. It's not coincidental that all mail-order nurseries dig, pot, and ship their trees and bushes in early spring. That's the time immediately following a plant's dormant period and preceding its new growth spurt when it puts out massive amounts of new roots. Some nurseries dig and ship trees in fall, too, after the growth has slowed but before the dormant period begins. Experience has shown, though, that fewer transplanting casualties occur with spring transplants. Not one to buck the odds, I do most of my foraging early in the calendar year although I have dug trees with various degrees of success all year long. If you're a beginning forager, though, you should stick to those first warm months of the year.

Unless you're an excellent planner and organizer (or an experienced backwoodsman), there is a problem when foraging for trees in spring: It's hard telling a 9-inch leafless elm from a 9-inch leafless maple. Many times, I've scoured the woods for a certain species of tree only to find some months later a complete surprise sitting in my living room. If you're a gambler, you know there's a way to beat the odds in just about every area of life — no less so in collecting trees in early spring. But you'll need to think ahead.

If you scout out the trees of your choice in early fall, in advance of leaf-shedding time, attach color-coded labels to the trees (orange for maple, red for ash, yellow for willow, etc.). The following spring, your only problem will be finding the labeled trees. Once that's done, you'll know exactly what type of trees you're digging with no surprises.

Another way to be relatively sure of the type of sapling you're unearthing is to check the species of mature trees around it. If you're in a thick stand of white birches, for example, you can be pretty sure you're not going to be digging up a shag-bark hickory. Of course, as long as the winds blow and the seeds fly, this method isn't foolproof. But it boosts the odds of getting the tree you desire to better than even.

Reducing the Shock

No matter when you dig trees to transplant indoors, you should keep in mind the plant's natural cycle. By imitating that cycle artificially, you'll improve your chances for success by reducing the degree of transplanting shock.

All home vegetable gardeners who start seedlings indoors know about the necessity of gradually *hardening off* young plants to reduce the likelihood of severe transplant shock before transplanting them outdoors. If a tomato seedling grown indoors in 74° F warmth is suddenly transplanted outside where the evenings dip to a nippy 40°F, the plant will quickly wither and die. But if the seedling is gradually hardened off — kept for a few days in a series of progressively cooler rooms — the amount of shock will be reduced and the seedling will have a better chance of surviving full-time outside.

Well, trees are plants, too, remember. And they're just as likely to suffer transplant shock as any other plant. Often, though, trees suffer an opposite kind of shock from that of most other types of seedlings. Whereas many plantlets are injured by being moved directly from a warm house to a cool garden, many trees are injured by the change from a cool yard to a warm, dry house. Under such circumstances, the tree's natural growth cycle is thrown for a loop. The plant suddenly bursts into bud, leafs out, and then begins sending out new root and limb growth. It's a tremendous strain on the tree's roots and source of energy, which it has shut down for the remainder of winter — a premature and unexpected strain that could be fatal.

I've seen trees suffer the opposite kind of shock, as well, thanks to the miracle age of technology in which we live. Trees yanked from the garden in the middle of their growing season (on, say, a 95°F August afternoon) and transplanted into an air-conditioned home can be terribly confused. It's similar to a person taking a scalding shower before jumping into a snowbank. You can imagine what the sudden drop in temperature does. For both the person and the trees!

To reduce the effect of transplant shock, keep the tree's natural growth cycle in mind. You can, for example, dig up an outdoor tree in midwinter, transplant it into a large pot, and then place it outside (preferably in a location sheltered from harsh northern exposures). Wrap the pot in burlap or straw to prevent serious damage to the roots from hard freezing in northern climes. Let the potted tree remain outside until the outside-inside temperature difference is minimal — 10 or 15 degrees. Then practice hardening off in reverse. (Perhaps *softening off* is a better term.)

First, move the pot to a cool room and then to a warmer one before finally placing it in its permanent indoor location. Allow from 7 to 10 days in each room for gradual adjustment. In that manner, you minimize the risk of loss from transplant shock and insufficient softening off and increase your chances for success. Remember to lightly water the plant occasionally during its dormancy (before new leaves start to show) to prevent the roots from drying out and dying. As the buds begin to swell and the sap starts to flow inside the tiny young trunk, the tree will require more water to sustain its growth. You'll find more information on proper watering techniques later in the book.

Breathing out, Breathing in

Whether you know it or not, transpiration is every gardener's mortal enemy. Master horticulturist Donald Wyman, in his book, *Wyman's Gardening Encyclopedia,* defines transpiration as "the physiological process by which water is given off by the leaves through the stomata, situated usually in both the lower and upper side of the leaf."

What that means in laymen's terms is that plants sweat. They lose water to the atmosphere continuously, which accounts for the fact that they never swell up like balloons even though the roots are constantly sending water up from the soil. This happens more on hot, windy days and less on cool, windless ones. If the plant's rate of transpiration is greater than its rate of absorption through its roots (as in the case of plants whose root systems are disturbed or mangled through transplanting), the plant withers and may die. How does a plant's rate of transpiration affect you as a collector? Very dramatically.

If you were to locate a grove of small maple trees and follow the identical procedures in digging up ten of them on a cool, rainy afternoon and ten more on a hot, sunny afternoon, you'd see graphic proof of the role transpiration plays in transplanting success. Whereas you'd have close to 100 percent success on the former day, your percentage might drop to 10 or 20 on the latter.

My most successful day of collecting trees came one cool, rainy, foggy morning in late May. I collected half a dozen young trees, including one that had been sitting bare roots exposed for several hours. I enclosed them all in plastic bags overnight and planted them the following morning, a less than advisable practice but unavoidable at the time. All trees survived without a single leaf loss. Not even minor droop! You'd swear they'd sprouted from seed right in those pots and had never been uprooted at all.

On the other hand, the least successful day of collecting I've ever been cursed with was a 92°F, bright, sunny June day. I dug up a dozen crab apple trees as an experiment (with a ball of earth clinging to each), sprayed them thoroughly with cool water, encased them quickly in plastic bags containing damp paper towels, and rushed them to the shade of my exposed back porch. Before they were potted, the leaves showed definite signs of droop. I sprayed them every few minutes while working, and then I watered the new transplants liberally. Finally, I encased the leaves in plastic bags tied with twist-ems around the trunks and punctured with pencil holes to aid air circulation.

The results of all my elaborate plans were disappointing. All twelve saplings died back to the ground. I had set out to see if I couldn't, through my own ingenuity, beat Mother Nature at her own game. But Nature, when she so chooses, is a more-than-worthy adversary.

Of course, the ideal — collecting trees and shrubs in the middle of a spring downpour — is something less than desirable. But at least you should confine your collecting forays to windless, cool, overcast days. Those are the days when a plant's transpiration rate is lowest — and your chance for success is highest.

The Right Size

There's another important consideration in collecting trees for transplanting indoors: size. Obviously, you can't transplant a year-old maple tree and let it grow to full size, not unless you use your entire basement for a pot and open a permanent skylight in your roof. But that doesn't mean you can't enjoy the beauty of a maple tree in your living room. In fact, depending upon how much work you want to invest and what sort of return you expect from your investment, you can use one of three ways to bring the giants of the tree world inside.

The first and easiest way is to transplant small young saplings and keep them indoors until they outgrow the pot, the room, or both. This usually happens within 2 or 3 years, at which time you can transplant the tree outdoors and start all over again with another young sapling for indoor growth. It's a never-ending transplanting cycle, of course, but it's ecologically sound and, in the long run, a gratifying experience. It's also an inexpensive way to improve your outdoor landscaping.

The second way you can bring that outdoor tree indoors is to make a bonsai specimen out of it. With regular maintenance, the tree may never grow taller than 9 or 10 inches, even if it lives to the age of 100. Bonsai is a little out of the realm of this book, though; we're more interested in large trees and shrubs than in miniature caricatures of them. If you're into bonsai, or would like to be, check the offerings on Google or at your local library. There are at least twenty good books currently in print that deal with the subject.

The last way to keep a tall grower indoors is what I most frequently do. You can allow the indoor tree to reach maximum proportions for the pot and the room. Then, instead of transferring the tree outdoors and starting all over again, you can unpot it, prune back both roots and top growth equally, and repot in the same container or a slightly smaller one. It's a bit of work, granted, and a little too messy to tackle right in the middle of the living room, but you'll have the satisfaction of knowing that, with a little yearly maintenance once maturity is reached, the tree you select for indoor growth today will still be gracing your home 20 years later.

Exactly how you go about pruning back both roots and foliage is the subject of a later chapter. For greatest success, be sure to read it before picking up a set of pruning shears.

Watch Out for Uninvited Guests!

There's no way on Earth to keep your trees from developing certain diseases or, more often, insect infestations from time to time. If you grow plants, you'd better resign yourself to that fact.

Many indoor gardeners think that because the plants they grow indoors will remain there, the plants are immune from attack. It's a nice thought but something less than realistic. What people forget is that all trees, unless propagated in someone's airtight basement, have been exposed to the outdoors at one time. And many collected and store-bought trees harbor pests that, when brought into the ideal growing conditions of your home, are all too willing to "share the wealth" with the rest of your plant collection.

Trees that you collect yourself, of course, are extremely likely to play host to various bugs. One maple tree I brought in several years ago underwent the closest scrutiny imaginable. I examined the bare branches and young trunk with a magnifying glass for any sign of insect or disease. Then I swabbed the sapling with a 50 percent concentration of alcohol just to be on the safe side. Finally, I put the potted tree under a cool shower to rinse away anything that was left that shouldn't have been there.

Within 2 months, the 9-inch maple budded, and then it burst into leaves. Some 3 weeks later, the leaves began turning brown along the edges. Along with the leaves, a hatch of whitefly eggs, which had been incubating in the soil brought in with the plant, had burst into "bloom." The insects had only to fly up a few inches to begin a life of feasting on the succulent juices flowing through the tender leaves' veins. I'd forgotten to wash

away the old soil and transplant the tree in sterilized soil or to treat the old soil with an insecticide that would have destroyed the whitefly eggs. A detail I haven't forgotten since. Luckily, I was quick enough to recognize the demons so that I saved the tree. Had I waited awhile longer, I would have lost the tree and forced the whitefly to seek new feeding grounds on the other plants and trees in my collection!

Besides taking the direct route of infiltration, pests and disease can enter the home, quite literally, on a breath of fresh air. Each time you open a door or crack a window, microscopic spores and eggs enter on a breeze. They float around the room until they find a suitable place to land. If they happen to wind up on the kitchen floor, they'll likely be mopped up and poured down the drain. But if they land on your beautiful 8-foot *Schefflera*, oh, brother! In a sunny, enclosed, constantly warm environment free from natural predators, pests such as mealybugs, aphids, and spider mites can grow wild!

What can you do to protect your highly susceptible trees and shrubs from infestation or to treat them to eliminate pests once they strike? We'll go into that in detail later in the book.

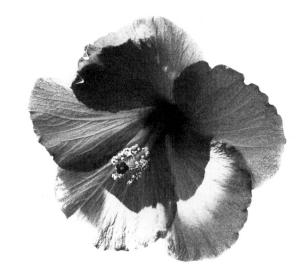

Chapter Six:

Soil: Preparing for Action

So YOU'VE GONE OUT and invested in the tree of your dreams to grace your living room. Or you've dug up a real beauty from the wild that's sure to look just right in your den. Where do you go from here?

There are several steps to follow in preparing to plant an indoor tree before you can begin enjoying the fruits of your labor. They include selecting a suitable pot, preparing the growing medium, and pruning the plant and its roots (yes, really). None of these steps is especially difficult or time-consuming, but each is crucial to the plant's healthy growth and development once you heel it into the pot.

Selecting an Appropriate Container

One of the joys of indoor gardening is the vast selection of containers available.

There's literally a look for every décor. Some pots are made expressly for plants, of course, while others are actually intended for different purposes. They are made from stone (either hand- or machine-carved), clay, wood, metal, plastic, or glass. Suitable containers also come in all kinds of shapes: standard flowerpots, cylindrical, spherical, square, oval, or rectangular pots, plus all sorts of irregularly shaped containers. There are many colors, raised textural patterns, and decorative finishes, from sandblast rough to glistening-chrome smooth.

Where to Find the Right One

Before considering where to look for containers large enough to hold your indoor trees and shrubs, you should first realize what you'll need in order to house your plants. Don't think only in terms of whatever pots your nursery or garden center sells. Sure, those may make excellent planters. But they're also expensive, especially when 12 inches or larger.

So, where can you find less expensive planters? Check out your local dollar store or building center. You might be amazed at their number of large watertight containers, ranging from laundry baskets and hampers to wash buckets and trash cans (both office size and backyard size). They could make excellent planters with a little painting, masking, or even as is. Or, if you're handy working with wood, you can cut some slats to the right size and attach them to the outside of your inexpensive container, turning it into a natural-looking work of art.

If you live near a junkyard, forget your pride and take a trip out there. For a few bucks or less, you should be able to find some real bargain planters. Don't look too interested in the merchandise, of course, and don't be afraid to dicker with the dealer.

If you live in a larger town or city, you probably have access to several container manufacturers. Check your telephone directory's yellow pages under "Cans." My town lists several manufacturers, one of whom advertises: "Cans — all types. In stock for immediate shipment, half a dozen or a truckload. Over five hundred sizes and styles, from 1/16 ounce to 55 gallons. Round, square, or rectangular. Free container guide and price list."

Also, check with any neighboring dairy farms or milk-processing plants. They just may have some old, ready-for-discard milk cans (five or ten gallons) that they'd be happy to part with for a few dollars. And scout around the antique stores and junk shops in the area. I bought an old milk can at one recently. After cutting off the top with a jigsaw, it took only a little scraping, sanding, and painting to end up with an excellent planter, both deep and wide enough for the tree I put in it. And the little strawberry begonias that cascaded down its side were an added bonus of color and texture.

The bottom line is that you don't have to pay an arm and a leg for a large planter if you use a little ingenuity and just a bit of elbow grease.

A special precautionary word about all-wood containers. A friend of mine used an old oak wine cask for a container to hold her 10-foot banana tree. The cask boasted plenty of room for the tree's roots, and it added a bit of rustic charm to her dining room. She placed the cask and tree just inside a large glass wall with a gorgeous southern exposure on some beautiful brown shag carpeting. You've probably guessed what's happened. Even though the cask once held liquid, all wood sweats. It's porous enough to allow some seepage of moisture over a period of time. If and when my friend ever decides to move the pot (which has been in the same location for several years now), she's not going to be very happy with the condition of the carpeting beneath it.

If you want to try your hand at using large wooden containers for planters, go right ahead. But first take some precautionary measures. Pick up a large, thick piece of acrylic sheeting to place beneath the planter. That way, the carpeting or your nice wooden floor will be protected from seepage. Or, easier and cheaper still, line the wooden container with two-mil plastic or heavier vinyl pond lining before adding the soil. You can buy the materials at most paint supply shops, nurseries, and building-supply centers.

As an alternative to lining your wooden planter, you can paint or spray it with a waterproof sealant, such as Drylok. Allow the sealer to dry, give it a second coat to be on the safe side, and you should be ready to go.

There is one potential drawback to using planters made of wood, clay, ceramic, and stone, and that's weight. If you plan on moving the filled planter around in order to catch the seasonally shifting rays of the sun, you'd be better off settling on a lightweight container made of plastic or poly resin. Either one is light enough and has the additional advantage of being easy to paint (with specially made plastic spray paints) so you can harmonize the planter's color with the room. And, while even

a large plastic pot filled with soil and a good-sized tree or shrub is far from light, at least you should be able to drag it across the room to wherever you want or enlist the aid of a couple of more people to pick it up and carry it to its new location. That's a much tougher job when your planter is made of heavy materials.

Size Does Matter

How large a pot should you use when planting a tree or shrub? Contrary to common sense, bigger is not always better. While various methods have been suggested for determining the proper pot size for a plant, I like the *one-third rule* best. Choose a pot whose diameter is one-third the height of the tree or shrub you're placing in it. If you're planting a 3-foot tree, choose a pot that's one-third that height, or 1 foot in diameter. A 6-foot tree requires a pot 2 feet in diameter and so on. This is just a rule of thumb, of course, and should be tempered by common sense. Don't put a 6-foot tree in a pot that's 2 feet in diameter and only 1 foot deep. And, if you're planting a low-growing shrub (perhaps 3 feet in height) with a 4-foot head (the width of the crown or top of the plant), you'd do better to select a pot nearly as large in diameter as the plant's crown or 3- to 4-feet in diameter.

The old guideline for naturally growing trees and shrubs (those growing outdoors) is that the plant's root spread is approximately as large as the crown spread. Thus, if you wanted your indoor tree or shrub to grow unencumbered by pot size, you'd select a container whose diameter is as wide as the plant's head at maturity. But a pot of such vast size would be hard to find, extremely expensive, and, of course, too large for most indoor settings. Most trees adapt well to a pot that has a diameter of one-third the plant's height. And plants in general are remarkably forgiving when it comes to having cramped quarters for their roots.

More Considerations When Choosing

Pot size isn't the only consideration you'll be faced with when matching your pots to your plants. Here are a few more elements to consider.

Container Scale. Scale is the relationship of the pot to its surroundings, as well as to the plants you place inside the pot. For a pleasing visual effect, your plants should be in proportion to the size of the container. Picture a fully grown yucca plant in a pot the size of a gallon milk jug. The scale would be entirely wrong, and the scene would look ridiculous. Conversely, a dwarf yew in a 36-inch pot would appear preposterous.

Also, when placing the potted plant, take into consideration the plant's

surroundings. Don't place a solitary 10-inch pot in the corner of a two-story solarium, or it will look a bit like a gnat on a hog's, umm, hind quarters. Contain single and smaller pots to small areas.

Container Color. The color of your containers should complement their surroundings. Choose a natural color that blends well with your indoor decor. Brightly colored pots in red, blue, and yellow do best as featured elements surrounded by other less vibrant pots. The eye will fall first on the splashy pots and gradually take in their neighbors. Remember that the plant should be the focus of attention; don't force it to compete with its container.

For the least intrusive pots, choose natural, unglazed terra cotta or lightly textured pots in muted earth tones.

Container Grouping. Pay attention to the number of pots you have in any given area. A single pot set off all alone nearly always looks inconsequential or lost, stark by comparison to its surroundings. By grouping three or more pots together, you'll lend a more natural look to the area. An uneven number of pots, by the way, appears to the human eye to be more natural than an even number, which the brain conceives to be contrived or staged. A word to the wise.

In order not to appear too garish, avoid grouping together several pots of wildly varying colors, shapes, and sizes. One large terra cotta pot surrounded by two somewhat smaller pots of similar construction, for instance, would be ideal for most corners, atriums, or entryways to a home.

As you would with any decorator elements, group pots according to their size, placing the larger pots toward the rear of the grouping and the smaller pots toward the front and off to each side.

Container Style and Shape. Choose a container that suits the general style of your home or garden or the area where the container is to be placed. Is your home country casual? Select a pot that complements it. Is the pot to go into a room adorned with Oriental artifacts? A Far Eastern motif would work best. Is your home classically formal in its decor? A Grecian urn-style pot or something similarly ornate might work best.

Beware, however, when selecting a container with a sleek, sculpted profile to avoid impractical pots with narrow necks that make repotting nearly impossible without breaking open or cutting the pot in two.

Container Material. The material from which the pot is made influences not only the aesthetic appeal of the planting, but also the rigor with which your plants will grow. Common terra cotta, clay, or cement pots, for example, are porous, allowing the soil to dry out more rapidly; so watering must be done more frequently than when using a nonporous container made of plastic, metal, or resin or a pot that has a ceramic coating, which prevents transpiration and requires less watering.

Whatever size and style pots you choose, remember to match the planting to its environment. Pots and plants should work together aesthetically instead of fighting one another for attention, and the planted container should fit comfortably into its environment, whether indoors or out.

Oh, and one more thing. If you have cats, be prepared. They love potted plants! To them, indoor trees and shrubs make the most inviting litter boxes in the world.

To discourage your cats from digging around (and worse) in your large pots, cover the surface with crumpled aluminum foil (for a short-term deterrent), large stones (large enough so that the cats can't claw them out of the way when they want to urinate or defecate), or pine cones (which look great and can be left in place year-round). You can also glue several slats of thin wood together in a tic-tac-toe fashion and place the slats on the soil for an attractive addition that will keep your pets from getting to the soil below. Or simply cover the exposed soil with a planted ground cover that your cats can't dig up, like clover or baby's tears.

Preparing for Planting

With all that finally out of the way, you're ready to consider the next step to take before actually planting your tree or shrub. And that step involves choosing the proper soil.

Now, *soil* is a ubiquitous term for what you see when you first walk outside your back door (your concrete patio or wooden deck to the contrary). But for the indoor gardener, it means "growing medium." It could be soil — just like you have outdoors — but more likely it will be a combination of growing media mixed together and sterilized to provide the best possible environment in which indoor plants can grow. This soil is the basis for indoor plant life. If it's healthy, well-balanced, and nutrient-rich, your trees and shrubs will grow well. If it's rocky, imbalanced, and devoid of nutrients, your plants will suffer. Guaranteed!

Soil is one of several aspects of gardening in which the indoor gardener has an advantage over his backyard cousin. While the outdoor gardener spends years trying to alter or amend the soil on his property — and then forever toils at keeping the makeup of the earth just the way he wants it — the indoor gardener can obtain a soil mixture made to order for the specific requirements of each tree and shrub in his home. You can purchase a different type of soil for each of the plants in your home if you choose.

As with procuring trees, there are two ways you can acquire good potting soil: buy it from a nursery or garden center or collect it from outside. If you're on a strict budget or plan on using a lot of soil, you may want to collect it. A small bag of potting soil, which may cost $2 or $3, won't go far toward filling the size of pot required for a large tree or shrub.

Even if you don't own your own property, there's always some place to collect a bushel full of dirt. There are building excavation sites where the soil has been dug up to be carted away (check for permission first). Your city or town may own a landfill with soil that needs to be removed. Or you may have property-owning friends who would gladly share a little terra firma with you for the asking — and the digging and hauling, of course!

But before you plant your valuable trees and shrubs in native ground, there are a couple of steps you need to take for your own protection and that of your plants. A soil's makeup depends on the way the soil is arranged and of what it consists. To discover the texture of the soil you've collected, you can run a simple test.

Place a quarter cup of soil and enough water to cover it in a quart jar. Seal the jar tightly, and slosh the mixture around for thirty seconds. Let it settle for a few minutes, and then slosh it around again. Set the jar aside for a day or so until the water clears. Examine the results in good light. What do you see?

At the bottom of the jar, you should see various layers of materials. The very coarsest layer consists of sand and stones. Above that, you should see finer sand. Above that, there should be a layer of fine silt. Clay will top off the sediment, with organic matter floating to the top.

Analyzing Your Soil

Analyze the proportions of these ingredients. If the sediment is more than half sand, you have what's called a *light sandy soil*. If the sediment is more than half silt and includes hardly any clay, you have a *heavy silt soil*. If it's more than a quarter clay and has a large amount of silt, you have a *heavy clay soil*. If the sediment in the jar is about two-fifths sand, two-fifths silt, and one-fifth clay, you have struck gardeners' *nirvana*. You've found an ideally composed soil. It's called good, rich *loam*. Don't forget where you got it, because you'll be going back for more.

If you have really good loamy soil, you'll see plenty of twigs, grass, and other organic matter floating on top of the water. A lot of this material means that, when you use this soil, billions of bacteria will be slaving away to draw various salts and minerals from the soil and turn them into solutions that a plant's roots can absorb and utilize for growth. This floating organic matter is called *humus*, and you can rarely have too much of it.

To increase the amount of humus in the soil you have collected, you can add any *organic matter* — peat moss, leaf mold, rotted manure, sawdust, compost, grass clippings, or even kitchen vegetable waste. (Caution: don't include *any* animal by-products such as bones, egg shells, grease, or meat scraps, or you'll be begging for an infestation of maggots.)

To improve a light sandy soil, add plenty of humus. To improve a heavy silt soil or a heavy clay soil, add plenty of humus and up to one-third coarse sand (builder's sand), perlite, or vermiculite.

How much humus should you add? Generally, a good loamy soil should be at least one-eighth humus. At *least*. A good source of humus, if you're a property owner, is your lawn. The green clippings can be dried out and sterilized quickly in a 450°F oven and added to your soil. But *only* if you don't spray your lawn with chemical fungicides, insecticides, or herbicides that will linger in the clippings and be passed along to your newly potted plant to spread the chemical poisons to your plants and, through respiration, throughout your home.

Another source of humus available to nearly everyone is vegetable waste from the kitchen. Collect all those carrot tops, potato peels, and other fruit and vegetable cast-offs. Chop the ingredients into small bits with a blender or by hand, place the material in a 450°F oven for an hour (to kill off any nasty insect eggs, fungus, or bacteria) and add it to your soil.

Autumn leaves also make excellent humus. They, too, should be dried out in the oven to sterilize them before crumbling and mixing them into the soil. A rich, loamy soil? It's easy to obtain for *any* indoor gardener. You've no reason to be without it.

Testing Your Soil's pH

Another consideration when choosing a growing medium is soil *acidity*. That's the balance between acidity and alkalinity as measured on a pH scale, a mathematical determination expressing a soil's concentration of hydrogen ions. Luckily, you don't have to be a mathematician or a chemist to change the acidity-alkalinity balance of your soil when required.

And when will that be? Most likely when you plant trees or shrubs requiring a specific pH in which to grow. Some plants such as holly (*Ilex*) and azalea (*Rhododendron*) grow best in acidic or "sour" soil while others such as honeysuckle (*Abelia*) and boxwood (*Buxus*) prefer alkaline or "sweet" soil.

On the pH scale, the number 7 denotes a neutral or perfectly balanced condition, neither acid nor alkaline. Numbers below 7 denote acidity— the lower the number, the higher the acidity. Numbers above 7 show alkalinity— the higher the number, the higher the alkalinity. Nearly all plants grow best in a pH range of 4 to 9 on a scale of 0 to 14. Most plants will tolerate soil that is slightly more acidic or alkaline than their preferred range.

If you plan on using the same soil for all your shrubs and trees, it would be wise to test the soil's pH and keep it in the 6.5 to 7 range (only slightly acidic). You can buy an inexpensive pH soil testing kit from your garden supply center or over the Internet.

What damage will an unsuitable pH do to your plants? If your trees and shrubs have all the nutrients they require, but the plants still show signs of malnutrition, the culprit may be the soil pH. Frequently, yellow leaves are caused by the inability of the plant to absorb the iron that has been locked into the soil by excessive alkalinity (a high number on the pH scale). Even though there's plenty of iron there, the plant simply can't utilize it.

To remedy the problem, you can add acidity to the soil, thus neutralizing the alkalinity and lowering the scale to around 7. Work pine needles, peat moss, sawdust, leaf mold, or powdered sulfur at the rate of half a cup of sulfur per 9 cubic feet of medium loam into the soil. That should lower the pH level around one point on the scale.

To make an acidic soil more alkaline, add powdered lime (a gardener's best friend) at the rate specified on the package. Wood ashes or ground oyster shells also add alkalinity to soil.

After altering your soil's pH, always test it again to make sure you haven't over-reacted to the problem and added too much acid or alkali.

Using Sterile Soil

Another problem you should be aware of in collecting your own soil is its lack of cleanliness or *sterility*. One of the big benefits of using packaged, commercial soil is that it may be sterilized (if it is, the label will say so). Even at that, soil collected in the wild can be sterilized easily enough in your kitchen oven.

Why bother to sterilize the soil at all? If you would use it right from the garden, you're bringing all sorts of insects, eggs, disease spores, and weed seeds in with it. Outdoors, all these "guests" have natural predators to keep them in check. Indoors,

there are no birds, ladybugs, lacewings, wasps, and praying mantises to help you out — nor any beneficial parasites that live on and destroy harmful insects.

To sterilize your collected soil, pour it into a large baking pan, such as a disposable aluminum pan you can buy at the grocery store for a dollar or two. Place the pan in the oven. Set the temperature to 450°F and bake for about an hour. After that, your processed soil will be as free of insects, diseases, and weed seeds as any commercially sterilized soil you can buy.

When the soil is "done," allow it to cool before using it in pots. And please: No "finger testing" allowed! Soil baked in a 450°F oven gets pretty hot and stays that way for quite some time — hot enough to inflict a serious burn to your hand. Instead, test the temperature with a kitchen thermometer to tell when it's sufficiently cooled to use.

I prepare nearly all the soil I use for indoor plants, adding additional coarse sand, perlite, and humus whenever necessary, and I've never been disappointed with the results. The process is fun and a lot less expensive than buying potting soil. My basic soil recipe includes around 25 percent topsoil (garden soil), 25 percent humus, and 50 percent coarse sand. For moisture-loving plants, I add a handful of humus to help retain moisture throughout the soil where the roots have access to it.

One last note about sterilizing soil in your kitchen oven: the smell from the decomposing debris is, uhh, "unique." It's earthy to say the least. If you're not sure you can live with that until the aroma dissipates, consider baking your soil on an outdoor grill.

Providing Adequate Drainage

Drainage is another variable with which you must be concerned — both in collected and purchased soils. In the wild, Mother Nature naturally provides adequate drainage for her trees and shrubs. You aren't quite so lucky. Yet, trees require good drainage so that their roots don't sit in a potful of soggy slush. That situation — called, coincidentally enough, *drowning* — can destroy roots and damage or even kill the plant in time.

The easiest and best way to provide drainage for your plants is to put them in pots drilled with drainage holes. Then simply match a saucer to the pot and — as with that small African violet growing on your kitchen windowsill — you're set to go.

But if you took seriously all that talk about finding and using containers not originally intended to hold your plants, you may say: "Ah-hah! A contradiction. I've been had!" Well, not really. There are at least two ways to provide drainage for plants in containers not already equipped with drain holes.

The easiest is not, unfortunately, the best. It consists of placing 2 to 6 inches of coarse stone or gravel in the bottom of the pot to provide a space for excess water to drain away from the plant's roots. Cover the gravel with cheesecloth or fiberglass screening before filling with soil to prevent the soil from filtering down into the stone with each watering and clogging up the drainage area.

In theory, then, as you water, the excess liquid flows into the gravel well at the base of the container below the roots and eventually evaporates. In *theory*. But problems arise if you add more water than the drainage well can hold. In that event, the water will begin getting wicked up into the soil where it can cause decaying roots, threatening the entire plant.

In such instances, you'll need to water carefully. The kicker, though, is that you can't ever be certain that you're not overwatering because you can't see what's going on in the bottom of the pot; you can only guess.

A more effective way of providing a well to drain off excess water is the "pot-within-a-pot" method. Start with a decorative, sealed container (no drainage hole). Add several inches of drainage material in the bottom. Then plant your tree or shrub in a second slightly smaller pot equipped with a drainage hole. Place the planted pot inside the decorative container. Voila! A pot-within-a-pot.

Of course, you'll still have to check from time to time to make sure the water from the planted pot hasn't leached into the pebbles in the decorative pot to a point high enough so that it's being reabsorbed into the planted pot's soil, endangering the roots. When the water reaches that height, you'll have to lift out the planted pot, empty the water at the bottom of the decorative container, and replace the planted pot. If the size and weight of the planted pot prevents you from lifting the container, you may be able to wick up the excess water from the decorative container with a towel, or you can use a wet/dry vacuum.

So, whether or not you decide to buy your containers and soil or get a little more creative in repurposing what already exists, is up to you. Either way, once you have your pot on hand and the growing medium ready to go, you're close to filling your home with health-giving trees and shrubs. Next up: Planting your trees and shrubs.

Science Says

Soil is the lifeblood of nearly all plants. It serves several functions, all designed to support robust plant growth by providing:

Anchorage. Root systems extend outward and/or downward through soil, thereby stabilizing your plant's top growth.

Oxygen. The microscopic spaces among the soil particles contain air that provides oxygen that the plant's living cells (including root cells) use to break down sugars and release the energy needed to live and grow.

Water. The spaces among soil particles also hold water, which is absorbed by and moves upward through the plants. This water cools plants as it evaporates off the leaves and other tissues, carries essential nutrients into plants, helps maintain proper cell size so that plants don't wilt and die, and serves as raw material for photosynthesis, the process by which plants capture light energy and store it in the form of sugars for later use.

Temperature modification. Soil insulates roots from dramatic fluctuations in temperature, particularly important during excessively hot or cold days.

Nutrients. Soil supplies the nutrients that we add in the form of plant food. The roots of a plant are particularly critical to your plants' overall health and development. One reason for that is the *rhizosphere*, the thin zone of soil surrounding your plant's root mass. The rhizosphere differs from the rest of the soil in that it often supports specific and unique organisms. For instance, certain fungi live together with roots to their mutual benefit; these *mycorrhizal relationships* provide the fungi with a place to live while the fungi assist in the plant's water and nutrient uptake. Similarly, some *nitrogen-fixing bacteria* grow together with certain plants, including many legumes (members of the bean family). The bacteria convert atmospheric nitrogen into forms that can be used by their host plants. When the host plant dies, the nitrogen compounds released during the decomposition process are available to the next crop. Any mutually beneficial relationship between two dissimilar organisms is called a *symbiosis*.[1]

Desirable Soil Qualities

Since container-grown plants are limited in the amount of soil mixture they have available to them, it's important to use the best quality planting medium possible. It should have several characteristics common to all good media, according to the North Carolina State Extension.

- **Permeability:** Necessary for air and water to penetrate the pore spaces to reach the roots.
- **Water-holding capacity:** High quantities of organic matter, smaller particle sizes, and smaller pore spaces increase a soil's water retention ability.

- **Drainage:** Larger particle sizes and pore spaces allow water to drain well.
- **Aeration:** Large particles and organic matter create air space that provides oxygen necessary for the roots to absorb for overall plant growth.
- **Weight:** The lighter the mix, the easier to move the container. Also, lighter mixes are symbolic of less bulkiness and more air space in the media.
- **Fertility:** Nutrients necessary for healthy plant growth.
- **Pasteurization:** A mix that has been exposed to heat to remove most weed seeds, insects and larvae, and diseases.[2]

Water, an Important Key

Water is an amazing vital requirement of plants because it's a "universal solvent" that dissolves more substances than any other single liquid known to man. It's also a renewable natural resource. It exists in nature as a solid, a liquid, and a gas. Its molecules *cohere*, or stick together to one another, and *adhere*, or stick to other surfaces. That gives water its ability to reach the top of the tallest trees. It has a high latent heat, which means that it *releases* a large burst of energy when it passes from solid to liquid and from liquid to gas. And, when it passes from gas to liquid and from liquid to solid, it *absorbs* a large burst of energy. Gardeners reap the benefits of all these attributes.

A soil's ability to hold water is called its *water-holding capacity*. Heavy clay soils have a high water-holding capacity while sandy soils have a low water-holding capacity. As a soil's pore space is filled with water, the soil becomes saturated. Then, the water gradually drains downward, and the amount of water remaining in the soil against the force of gravity is called the soil's *field capacity*. Clay-heavy soils drain much more slowly than sandy soils. Loamy soils reach their field capacity two to three days after a soaking watering. If no more water is added, the soil continues to dry out.

Of course, plants take up some of the water, and some water moves upward in the soil to evaporate from the surface. Eventually, a soil may become dry enough to reach its *permanent wilting percentage*, the point at which a plant wilts so severely that it cannot recover. At the point of permanent wilting percentage, the amount of *available water* (water that remains available to the plant) is gone, and the only water that remains in the soil is so tightly bound to soil particles that plants cannot access it and die.[3]

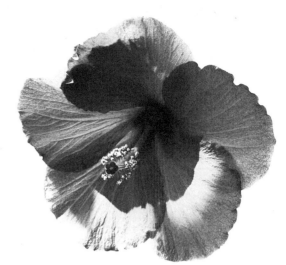

Chapter Seven:

Planting Your Indoor Trees and Shrubs

I F YOU BUY YOUR TREES AND SHRUBS from a local nursery or a mail-order house, the plants will arrive at your home in one of three conditions: potted, balled, or bare root (usually wrapped in damp paper or plastic for protection).

If the plant's roots are balled in burlap, you won't have any root pruning to worry about. You'll plant the tree, burlap and all, and hope the guys who wrapped it initially knew what they were doing. Once you plant it, look for any broken or dead branches and clip them back to a growing limb or bud. We'll discuss pruning in more detail later.

If the plant is potted in a plastic container, water it lightly and wait for 30 minutes. Then place your hand against the soil with your fingers straddling the main trunk and turn the pot over. Lift the pot off the root ball. Shake it gently if it's stubborn. If you're lucky, the root ball will slide out freely. If not, take a pair of tin snips or heavy-duty cutters or even a sharp knife and make a slit down one side of the pot to the bottom. Do the same on the opposite side of the pot. Don't cut too far into the dirt, or you may damage some of the roots. Once you've slit the plastic, you can carefully peel the pot back and remove the tree by banging what's left of the pot on a hard surface and then turning it upside down. Hold your hand on top of the soil where the trunk meets the earth so that, when the pot falls away, you have a good grip on the plant. The tree should slip out of the pot with little trouble or loss of dirt.

Once the tree is unpotted, check for any roots that are extending from the dirt and, with a pair of sharp pruning shears, cut away any broken or obviously dead roots. Be careful not to knock off any more dirt than necessary.

On bare-root stock (usually wrapped lightly in excelsior or shredded paper), keep the roots damp until planting time by soaking them thoroughly. After pulling back the excelsior and exposing the roots, prune back any broken or dead roots. If the operation takes more than a minute or two, dunk the roots periodically in a bucket of water. Exposure to air for even a couple of minutes may cause delicate, fibrous feeder roots to dry out and affect the plant's chances for survival.

Once the root pruning is complete, you're ready to plant.

Planting Your New Acquisitions

Planting trees and shrubs is hardly one of the world's more difficult tasks. It is a little more involved than stuffing the roots into a potful of dirt and waiting for the plant to shoot up. Prior to planting, you should have completed several steps. Let's check them out.

First, you selected and prepared a suitable container. Then you readied the soil, either the store-bought variety or the home-created stuff; you collected drainage gravel if necessary, and you made sure whatever you collected or bought was sterilized. Finally, you pruned away any broken or dead roots, being sure to keep the root mass damp while working.

If you did all that, you now have before you a soggy root mass, a bulky pot, what seems to be a ton and a half of soil, some gravel for drainage, and dirty fingernails. All

five elements go together like chicken and dumplings at a Sunday afternoon social.

Start by placing several inches of gravel in the bottom of the container as discussed previously. (Even if the container has drain holes, the gravel is a good idea.) Cover the stones with cheesecloth or fiberglass screening and fill the pot around one-third with dirt. What you do next depends upon how the plant arrived.

Balled Plant

Take the plant and place the root ball inside the pot, leaving the burlap in place. If you'd like, you can slit the burlap (lightly, now!) vertically in several locations to help the roots escape their confines. Make sure that the crown of the plant — the spot where the trunk meets the roots — is an inch or so below the lip of the pot. If the plant sits too high, remove some of the dirt beneath the root ball. If it sits too low, add some soil beneath the root ball to bring the crown up to the right height.

Once the plant is situated properly in its new home, center it and begin adding soil a little at a time. Tamp the soil down to remove any air pockets as you go. You've added enough when the soil comes to a point barely below the plant's crown. Never bury the crown beneath the soil, or you'll risk rotting the crown and killing the plant.

Finally, water lightly but thoroughly, which means until the water begins to seep out of the pot's drainage hole. That's when you know you're done. Then position the pot wherever you'd like it to be, and step back to admire your work.

Bare-root Plant

Remove most of the excelsior or shredded paper or moss around the roots, spray the roots lightly so they don't dry out while you're working, and gently spread them out into a fan-like splay. Position the plant atop the soil. Again, if the plant is too low, add more soil beneath the roots. If it's too high, take some soil out.

With the plant roughly centered in the pot and the roots spread out, begin adding soil a little at a time, tamping it down with your fingers or palms as you go. Stop when you've reached a point just below the plant's crown. Water lightly but thoroughly.

Potted Plant

Carefully lift the plant up by its root ball and peel away some of the soil clinging to the roots. The goal is to open up the roots so that they can grow freely once transplanted in their new home, but not to pull on them hard enough to damage or break them. Use your open fingers like a comb, gently raking the soil to separate as many of the roots as practical. Once you've opened up the root mass, set the plant inside the prepared pot and double-check for space. The roots should have enough room so that they don't touch the sides of the pot. If they do, you'll need to prepare a larger pot, making sure to keep the roots moist while you search.

Note: Occasionally you'll run into a plant whose root mass is so tightly interwoven that it's impossible to penetrate with your fingers. If that's the case, take a sharp knife and make several inch-deep slits in the root ball near the bottom. Then, work your fingers into the soil into the slits and gently pull apart some of the roots so they can begin growing freely once planted. If you plant a tightly woven root ball just as it is, there's a good chance the roots will continue growing in that confined space instead of spreading out into the potting soil, thus stifling the plant's growth and possibly killing it in time. So, as harsh as it may seems to cut into the root mass, it's preferable to do so whenever necessary.

Once the plant is situated in the right-sized pot, check for the height of the plant, adjusting the soil up or down as necessary until its crown comes to within 1 inch or so of the container's lip. Fill the pot with soil a little at a time, tamping it down as you go until you've reached a point just below the plant's crown. Water lightly but thoroughly.

If you haven't guessed by now, although one person can usually handle the job of planting just fine, two people can make everything go a little more smoothly. Especially in planting larger trees and shrubs, it's convenient to have an extra set of hands to hold the plant upright at the proper planting depth while you add soil and tamp it down to remove any air pockets that can dry out and damage the roots. Just remember that, as you tuck the soil into the various nooks and crannies and corners of the pot, you need to be gentle. This should be an easy operation, not a comedic duo featuring King Kong and Fay Wray.

By the way, no matter how often you plant trees and shrubs into containers, sooner or later you're going to situate the plant too low or too high in the pot, which will ultimately affect the height of the soil in the pot. Too low means you're losing valuable real estate that the plant could use for its root growth. Too high means you'll be overflowing the top every time you water the plant, messing the floor. Filling the tamped soil to within 1 inch of the container's lip is the perfect height.

If you do find you've made an error in judgment in situating the plant, simply remove some of the soil and reposition the roots until the plant is where it's supposed to be. Replace the soil, and you and your plant can live happily ever after.

Once you're finished planting, wipe the outside of the container with a clean cloth or sponge. Nothing looks less attractive than a healthy new plant in a container that looks as if it followed Bogey over the falls in the *African Queen*.

Finally, when everything else is finished, place your newly potted tree in a suitable location. Avoid exposing it to direct sunlight for several days until the plant has had an opportunity to recover from transplant shock — however slight it might be. After a few days, you can safely introduce it to direct sunlight a little at a time.

Science Says

Whenever repotting a plant, it's tempting to move it into a substantially larger pot so that you won't have to transplant it again in the near future. That's unwise. It's best to use a pot no more than one size larger than the plant's existing pot. In other words, you can move your plant up from a 4-inch to a 6-inch pot but not to an 8-inch or 10-inch pot. If you repot your plant into too large a container, the plant will utilize most of its energy toward sending out roots to fill the larger pot at the expense of creating new top growth.

By repotting into a container no more than one size up, you'll minimize the "stunted growth" period of the plant so that it can divide its energy more equally between the roots and the top growth, making everybody happy.

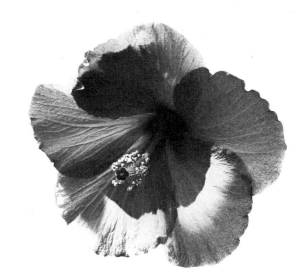

Chapter Eight:

Light, Water, and Humidity

Within the pages of the hundreds upon hundreds or even thousands of indoor plant books, booklets, and pamphlets in print today — not to mention the thousands of hours of video available on the Internet alone — you'll run across some false statements. Just as with the fake news that pervades our society, many of these statements are relatively harmless. Others aren't. I've seen numerous claims that the average indoor gardener can't start pine trees from seed to which I say — Nuts! Others warn against growing any plant in direct sun to which I say — Huh?

The point I'm making is this: No matter how good the advice in a particular book sounds, it must be tempered by your own experience, the experience of several other plant experts, and your plant's individual growing requirements. In this book, I tell you of my experiences and those of other acknowledged experts in the horticultural field. Fortunately, there are some universal truths about growing trees and shrubs indoors. Among the most important is that every plant needs three things to survive: light, water, and humidity.

Lighting Up

A plant shop owner and house-call specialist in Chicago claims that up to three-quarters of the ailing plants he visits every year would be healthy if their owners realized how important light is to a plant's growth and well-being. He finds that most people overestimate the amount of natural light available in certain areas or rooms. What they describe to him as "bright indirect light" often turns out to be very low light capable of sustaining few plants outside of *Philodendrons, Dieffenbachia,* and some ferns.

How does this lighting expert know that his customers are overestimating the light in their homes and offices? He asks them to evaluate the lighting and follows up by checking out their estimates with a light meter, which he uses to measure every area of available light in foot-candle power. Most people are amazed to discover how little light actually exists in a room they considered "bright."

What many people fail to realize is that what's bright to us is not necessarily bright to plants. Many plants grow naturally in full, direct sunlight outdoors. That's far more light — especially in summer — than human beings could possibly endure fourteen or sixteen hours a day. Think of what basking by the pool in direct summer sun would do to you in a few hours — let alone days, weeks, months, and years! It's no wonder people have a tendency to overestimate brightness within their own homes.

Yet, unless you're a photographer used to taking light-meter readings and translating them to relatively easy-to-understand figures, the best you can hope for is a simple approximation of indoor brightness. But with some facts in mind, the process becomes less of a guessing game and more of an art.

Know Your Home's Exposures

I'm continually amazed at how many indoor gardeners fail to know what their homes' various exposures are or even

what different exposures mean for their plants. Most streets in neighborhoods throughout North America are arranged in grids running north and south, east and west. That means most homes have northern, southern, eastern, and western exposures, depending upon the way you're facing as you look out a window.

If you're looking south, that window is said to have a southern exposure. If you're looking east, it has an eastern exposure, and so forth. Windows with a southern exposure have the brightest light exposure each day throughout the year. Both eastern and western exposures receive light about half the day and have moderate light exposures. (Beware, though, that western exposures receive the rays of the afternoon sun which are somewhat stronger than the morning rays that illuminate eastern exposures, so the two aren't absolutely comparable.) A northern exposure receives the least amount of direct sunlight and is said to be a low light exposure.

This simple fact of exposure is critical to know because different trees and shrubs need different amounts of light, depending upon their natural growing conditions. If you know your home's exposures, you can position your plants throughout the house for their maximum benefit.

Which spot in your home offers the greatest concentration of light? It's the southern exposure, as we said. However, the light at that south-facing window is strongest nearest the window or door pane. If the plant is set away from the glass only 3 feet, the light the foliage receives is cut in half! That means a plant set back from the window, even though in a room with a southern exposure, is actually getting much less than full sun — perhaps the equivalent of an eastern or western exposure! If the plant needs the maximum sun of a full southern exposure, that lack of light will likely stunt its growth.

Similarly, a plant that requires the moderate light of an eastern or western exposure isn't getting it if it's set back 3 or 4 feet from an east- or west-facing pane. And pity the poor plant situated several feet back from a weak northern exposure! The light that plant receives is practically non-existent. Only the most shade-loving plants will survive in a situation such as that.

Let's Get Serious

Scientists have a way of comparing different amounts of light. They use a unit of measurement called a *foot-candle* to describe the amount of illumination from any given source. One foot-candle is said to be equivalent to the amount of light cast on an object by one candle burning at a distance of 1 foot. Clever, huh?

But here's something I'll bet you couldn't have guessed. To get an idea of

the wide variance of lighting conditions in comparative indoor situations, check out this chart showing how much relative light is available on average under these conditions.

Indoors	Foot-candles Required
Housecleaning	5
Reading or Writing	20
Ironing or Sewing	40
Shop Work	40
Hotels	
Dining Room Eating	5–10
Lobby Registration	20
Offices	
Conference Room Meetings	30
Typing	50
Stores	
Warehousing	50
Shopping	100–200

Now, in comparison, take a look at the next chart, which shows the average amount of light available outdoors on various days.

Outdoors	Foot-candles Available
Cloudy Winter Day	2,000
Sunny Summer Day	10,000

What these charts tell us is that, even on the most overcast day, the light outside is still far greater than that available to plants indoors under average home lighting conditions. That's why people frequently overestimate their indoor lighting availability — often with a dire outcome for their plants.

So how does a plant suffer when it gets too little light? Does it get eyestrain? Does it get cranky? Actually, a plant shows no signs at all of trouble from too little light, at first. Plants can live for fairly long periods of time off the reserve food supplies stored in their roots without having to rely on light to manufacture food within their leaves. Eventually, though, that reserve gets used up. Without being able to manufacture its own food through the remarkably complex process of photosynthesis, the plant becomes spindly and sparse. Its new leaves become larger (in an effort to help the plant catch more of the elusive light per leaf) but fewer between. The stem stretches vainly toward whatever minimal source of light it detects. Finally, the lower leaves begin dying off from starvation.

In the case of flowering trees and shrubs, the plants may receive enough light to maintain sufficient foliar growth but not enough to produce flowers or set fruit.

The entire process may take as long as a year or more, but all light-starved plants will grow sickly and eventually die. The cure, of course, is to give them more light gradually so that they can begin manufacturing food full-force again. A *Ficus benjamina* that received poor light for several months and is suddenly thrust into direct, strong exposure will suffer as much as if it had continued on its light-starvation diet. The key to increasing a plant's light absorption is to give it more light gradually, so that it has time to adapt its system to the additional stimulus.

A few other factors also help determine how much light a plant receives. Dirt on the window, for example, greatly reduces the amount of light entering a room. To give a plant all the available light possible, especially in northern exposures where light is limited the most, be sure to keep the windows clean inside and out.

Draperies and curtains, blinds, and other window coverings also reduce the amount of light entering a room. Even if the coverings are open, they likely reduce the size of the glass that's exposed to the light.

Adding More Light

Fortunately, there are several ways to increase the light in your home, even if you live in a cave. Thanks to good old American ingenuity (and the current boom in houseplants), a wide range of incandescent, fluorescent, and LED grow lights has flooded the market. For as little as $3, you can replace the bulb in a living room lamp with the equivalent of a 60-watt grow lamp to subsidize the natural light your plants receive. Or, for hundreds of dollars, you can have installed an elaborate and mazelike system of track lighting so you can move the lights to exactly where you want to place your plants.

On one recent trip to my friendly home center, I bought a 150-watt incandescent grow light for $4 and a porcelain-based reflector socket (recommended because of the high heat that grow lights throw off) for under $6. The total with tax was less than $10. More recently, I found a twin-head (two lamps) LED fixture that clamps onto the top of a pot and can be pointed anywhere light is needed most — all for less than $20, including postage and delivery!

Of course, grow lights aren't the only answer to a dark-home. If you have a spot begging for a tree but there's no electrical outlet nearby, you can benefit from a design trick used by plant specialists. Get two identical plants, say *Schefflera*, and put one in the darker area and the other in a well-lighted spot more suited to its needs. After a month or two, swap out the plants, moving the sunny plant into the shade and the shaded plant into the sun — gradually, though. Continuing in that manner, you can keep both *Scheffs* relatively healthy and happy and make everyone in the family admire your green thumb.

In order to ease the pain of moving two large tubs filled with *Scheffs* around like a couple of potted begonias, pick up a pair of heavy-duty trivets. Or, instead of buying them, make them yourself if you're reasonably handy. They also prove useful when wintering plants in a cool place such as the garage or cellar or when over-summering your plants outdoors on the patio. When moving day arrives, just roll the plants to their new locations.

Reflecting Light

Another way of increasing the exposure of your trees and shrubs to more light is to multiply the intensity of the existing light through reflection. In a typical room, light enters once, and whatever the plants fail to catch is absorbed by walls, furniture, and draperies. But if the light is reflected off the walls and back toward the plants, your trees and shrubs will have a second chance at snaring those health-generating rays. In effect, the light entering the room does double duty.

You can reflect light in a room by adding mirrors or mirror tiles to one or more of the walls or by repainting the room in a reflective white or other light color.

"One of the most direct ways to use mirrors to increase sunlight in a room is to place mirrors on walls opposite the window," according to an article by Kathy Adams on SFGate. "For instance, if your family room or den has only one small window and some sunlight shines through, place a mirror on the wall directly opposite the window, so inbound sunlight reflects back into the room, magnifying the effect. If there is no wall directly opposite the window, place a mirror on an adjacent wall far enough away from the window that you can see the window reflected in the mirror."[1]

How can you tell if all your efforts are now giving your plants too much light? If you water them normally but the leaves begin to turn brown, get brittle, and fall off, that's a sign. Don't ignore it. For most trees and shrubs, too much light — especially direct southern exposure — can be every bit as damaging as too little. To remedy the situation, cut back on the amount of artificial light showering the foliage or move the affected plants back from their natural source of light.

Water

An associate of mine once bought a stately *Dracaena marginata* in a 10-inch pot. The plant stood over 4 feet tall and boasted a head of lush green foliage. He was justifiably proud of his acquisition, and he gave it a prominent showplace near a southern exposure in the living room. It was his first experience with growing trees indoors.

Within 2 months, several of the lower fronds grew pale and turned yellow before finally falling off. Before long, the entire plant drooped. His diagnosis: the plant was dying of thirst because he hadn't been watering it enough.

So, he boosted his watering program from once a week to every 4 days, then every 3. In between watering, he misted the plant daily. Nothing seemed to help.

Finally, he called for advice.

Well, I knew at a glance what the trouble was. The fronds were puffy and swollen. The fallen growth was banana yellow. The soil was saturated. The roots below the surface were undoubtedly beginning to rot. The diagnosis: overwateritis!

Often, plants that have been overwatered aren't diagnosed until too late. By then, they're dead, their roots drowned by the very life-sustaining element so necessary to their health. This *Dracaena marginata* survived and is now growing as if nothing had ever been wrong. But in order to heal itself, it required transplanting into a drier soil and 3 weeks without any water whatsoever to allow the roots to heal. Now, it receives a healthy watering about twice a month. That's a far cry from every three or four days!

My friend was one of many who believe plants die only from too little water, never too much. In fact, the contrary is true. More plants by far die from overwatering than from underwatering. Too much moisture prevents the tiny hair-like fibrous roots from obtaining the air they need to survive. As a result, the roots swell, weaken, and begin to decay. Thus damaged, they're incapable of supplying the plant with the nutrients so necessary for its life. In effect, first the plant drowns, and then it starves.

While it's true that many small houseplants, especially those planted in 3- or 4-inch clay pots, dry out quickly and thus require frequent watering, most people don't realize just how much moisture a large pot filled with rich loamy soil can hold, or for how long. On top of that, plastic or glazed ceramic pots — the types so many trees and shrubs are planted in these days — prevent evaporation better than clay or wooden pots.

So, that raises the question: How often should you water a large tree or shrub? Unfortunately, there's no watering timetable for any houseplant. The only sensible and effective way of determining when a plant needs watering is via the touch test. In small-to-moderate-sized pots, drill your finger into the soil at least down to the first knuckle (about 1 inch). If the soil feels relatively dry and your finger comes out with little or no soil clinging to it, reach for the watering can. If the soil feels moist and your finger emerges with moist particles of soil clinging to it, wait another day or two and test it again.

Of course, you have to temper the test with common sense. With larger pots, you'll need to dig that finger in deeper to determine the water situation. Remember that the soil in a pot dries out first at the surface and then gradually toward the bottom where the plant's roots are concentrated. If the soil on top feels dry to the touch, that doesn't mean the earth isn't saturated a couple of inches below the surface. Remember: It's what's below that counts.

Too Much or Not Enough?

If you find your favorite plant turning strange shades of every color except green, the question is, "Am I overwatering or underwatering?"

Generally speaking, if the leaves turn from green to a dry crackly brown, the plant isn't receiving enough water. If you water regularly, you may not be thoroughly saturating the soil between waterings, allowing the soil below the surface to remain dried out. Make sure the water runs from the drain holes in the bottom of the pot before assuming the plant has had enough.

On the other hand, if the leaves turn from green directly to yellow and begin to fall off, you're overwatering. Cut back on your watering scheduling immediately. If the plant shows little sign of improving within a few days, it may need a pruning job (both leaves and roots) and repotting in fresh dry soil. All you can do then is wait. And cut down on trips to the watering can!

After a few weeks of experience with touch-testing, most indoor gardeners get the hang of it. As with so many things in life, experience is the best — in fact, the only — teacher here. For those with weak fingers or an aversion to dirt, several manufacturers sell moisture meters with a metallic prod that you stick into the earth. The prod is attached to a dial that shows the relative degree of moisture in the soil. When it reads "dry," you water.

Of course, the rule that you should allow your trees and shrubs to dry out somewhat between watering is a good one for most plants, but it's only a generalization. Some plants require continuously moist soil, although they're certainly in the minority. Cranberry bushes, for example, prefer highly acidic, constantly moist soil. Other plants that prefer to remain on the damp side between waterings are discussed in later chapters.

How Much Is Enough?

There's no magic formula by which you can determine how much water is needed by a particular species of plant in a pot of a certain size. But there is a non-magic rule of thumb that says: water thoroughly. Notice, not regularly but thoroughly. A person who gives his palm tree a few ounces of water every other day is actually

killing it. While he's moistening the surface and encouraging surface-root growth, he's neglecting the deep-down soil and discouraging deep-root growth. The first time the surface soil dries out even for a day or two, all those surface roots will dry out, wither, and die right along with the deeper-running roots. There will no longer be enough healthy roots to sustain the plant through the drought.

But how does one tell when the soil is saturated from top to bottom? The only sure way is to water until you see the excess running out of the pot's drainage hole. The amount of that water will depend on the location of the plant in the home or office (plants dry out more quickly in warm, direct sunlight than they do in shade), as well as the growth pattern of the plant, the composition of the soil, the time of year, and even the material from which the pot is made.

Another question that frequently arises is whether to use tap water or filtered or distilled water. The answer is that tap water is usually fine. If you live in an area where the water is heavily chlorinated, though, allow a jug or two to sit out uncovered overnight to help oxidize, or neutralize, the chlorine.

Also, I've heard that soft water — the kind that's treated by a home water softener before it reaches your taps — is bad for plants. I've never had anything I know of die because of soft water. If you'd prefer not to take chances, draw your plants' water from the outside spigot, which is usually unsoftened for the sake of economy. Bring the water inside and let it warm to room temperature before using it on your plants. In fact, you should never use cold water that can shock a plant beyond recovery.

Humidity

There's never enough moisture in the air of a home to suit most plants. Not naturally, at least. In winter, especially in northern areas, there's hardly enough humidity to suit our needs. For us, that means dry, scratchy throats and swollen, blocked sinus passages. And plants take dryness even harder!

Without sufficient moisture, the leaves of trees and shrubs lose their brilliant leathery look. Their tips and edges may turn brownish yellow; minor cuts and scrapes may fail to heal quickly if at all.

I know from experience that, on frigid nights, the hygrometer will dip as low as 25 percent. That kind of relative humidity is extremely uncomfortable to humans and potentially deadly to plants, particularly exotic tropical plants that are acclimated to 80 or 90 percent relative humidity. Growing plants such as those becomes an all-out war.

The big question, of course, is how to increase the humidity in your home.

When dealing with small potted plants, you can follow the instructions in those wonderful little books that advise you to fill a tray with pebbles, setting the plants in the tray, and keeping the pebbles half covered with water. The evaporating water from the tray provides a moist mini-atmosphere for the plants.

But how about when dealing with a potted *Zelkova* stuck amid nearly 200 pounds of soil or a towering fiddle-leaf fig or even a Norfolk Island pine? Then maintaining suitable humidity involves more than a tray of pebbles sitting in a bath full of water.

The most efficient (and costly) way of beating those "dry-house blues" is to install an automatic humidifier. You can set the dial at the degree of humidity you want, and the device does the rest. After all, for a thousand dollars or more, it should!

Other humidifiers work just as well on a smaller scale. Many manufacturers make single-room models holding up to 7 or 8 quarts of water. When the humidity drops to a certain point, the machine kicks into action, spewing moisture into the air. Prices for these portable models are considerably lower than for whole-house humidifiers, and most units are on wheels so they're easy to move around.

If you're opposed to spending money for any type of humidification system, don't give up the ship. You can still add humidity to your indoor trees, albeit on a plant-by-plant basis. Taking a tip from the pebble-and-tray people, you can spread a layer of peat moss on top of the soil and keep the moss damp by misting it daily. When you touch-test the soil for watering purposes, move the moss to one side before digging your finger into the dirt.

Another way of accomplishing the task is more labor-intensive but still an old standby. Pick up a spray bottle and fill it with filtered water. Spray your humidity-loving plants often, at least daily. For a few dollars more, you can purchase a power-spray mister: pull the trigger, and it pumps out an adjustable stream of cool mist until you release it. The spray will add moisture to the air immediately around the plant while keeping the plant's leaves cool and healthy.

How Hot Is Hot?

Okay, that's it for cool-weather humidity. But what do you do if your home's climate is too hot? Contrary to popular belief, hotter isn't necessarily better for plants. In fact, for most plants, heat without humidity is damaging. The average home — even one equipped with a central humidifier — simply can't provide sufficient moisture to prevent plants from drying out in a 75°F or 80°F room. Ideally (for the plants, that is), the indoor temperature should be

between 68°F and 70°F. It's easiest to humidify air at that temperature. For every degree of heat above that, an increasingly large volume of moisture is required to raise the humidity level a single point!

Note that, in your efforts to keep your home from becoming too hot, you shouldn't fall prey to the trap at the other end of the spectrum. Cool is good; cold is not. Be sure to keep all your most delicate tropical plants away from leaky windows and doors during the winter months and from powerful fans and air-conditioners throughout the summer.

How Are Things in Casablanca?

Aside from having a cute subhead, this section actually has a point. Indoor plants grow quite well in Casablanca, thank you very much, for several reasons. First, the heat. Second, the humidity. Third, those adorable ceiling fans that are once again the rage. They do more than look nice, especially where trees and shrubs are concerned. They keep the air moving. That's very important for nearly all indoor plants. By continuously providing the plants with lightly moving air, the fans keep the plants from overheating and drying out. The air also helps to discourage the formation of fungus and mold on damp soil. As a bonus, moving air dissuades those little nasties such as whitefly and aphids from attacking your plants.

Another even simpler way of aerating a room, as long as you don't live in the Sahara, is by opening the windows. Gentle summer breezes can do wonders for a plant's general health. Sometimes 21st-century man, in all his wisdom, tends to forget just how wise Mother Nature can be. And how simply effective she is.

Science Says

Everything — from plants and animals to people — depends on water for life. A plant's roots function like a water pump where the water acts as a solvent that conveys minerals and other nutrients from the roots to the leaves. The water then evaporates and falls back to the soil to repeat once more its function in the life cycle.

No water, no cycle, no life. That's what it's like in the wild, and the same applies to our indoor plants, although on a smaller scale. When there are a lot of indoor plants, a suitable indoor climate is created because the plants give off moisture, use carbon dioxide, and yield oxygen of benefit to one and all.

Water for Nutrition and Coolness

Plants use water to transport nutrients to every part of the plant, as we said. But they also use water to regulate their climatic environment, just as people do. A great deal of the water the plant sucks up is used to maintain the correct internal temperature. Plants perspire just as we do when it is too hot for us. They keep down their temperature by transpiring water through sweating.

The leaves of a sunflower outside, for example, sweat out as much water on a hot day as a person does, and a birch tree can suck up hundreds of gallons of water and emit cooling dampness between its leaves on a hot summer's day. If they don't have enough water (and air) to transpire, they dry out, wither, and die.

Water Affects a Plant's Appearance

Plants adjust to their location. The amount of precipitation and the water available to them help decide the plant's shape and appearance. Plants that grow in locations that go through very dry periods learn how to save water. They do so by developing water reservoirs in their leaves, stems, and tubers, while at the same time they have a thick outer skin that slows evaporation.

Plants that grow in areas with little rainfall develop incredible abilities to adapt. They often bear seeds that can wait for rain for months or even years to germinate. When it finally comes, the plants sprout everywhere. Water really is life!

Alkaline Water

In many places where the soil is alkaline, the water contains a great deal of calcium and is therefore not very suitable for indoor plants. Many plants can't tolerate so much calcium over a long period of time: just as hard water leaves unattractive "water marks" on pots, misting plants with hard water results in calcium spots on their leaves. The calcium in hard water can be neutralized by adding small quantities of sulfate of ammonia or by boiling the water so that the calcium precipitates out (cool it to room temperature before using).

Overwatering

Far too many plants die by drowning (overwatering) because people water them too often and too much. Not all plants have the same water requirements. Generally, though, it's better to water at intervals of several days (or once or twice a week) as opposed to watering a little each day. But always check the soil before watering.

Too much water in the soil makes it sodden and incapable of supporting life. The water forces all necessary oxygen from the soil, and the roots begin to rot. Soon, the plant collapses. So, it important to adjust your watering schedule based upon the plants' needs.

Least Water in Darkest Months

Many plants have a rest period in the winter and need nearly no water at all — particularly if they are being kept cool, as in an unheated garage or basement. An exception are winter-flowering plants, such as azaleas, that require plenty of water to support their flower bud production. Know the yearly cycle of your plants and make watering adjustments to meet their needs. You'll find that watering gets easier the more you get to know your plants.

What You Can Do to Avoid Overwatering

1. Know your plants' specific needs. Do they like to be kept evenly moist or allowed to dry out some between waterings?

2. Put a finger in the soil to feel whether or not it's damp. If it is, there's no need to water. Of course, that doesn't tell you the condition of the soil toward the bottom of the pot, but if the surface soil is dry, chances are good the lower soil isn't saturated.

3. Always empty the saucer underneath the pot. Don't let the pot sit in a tray full of water for more than 20 or 30 minutes after watering.

4. Never give your plants little gulps of water. It's better to water thoroughly once a week than to give the plants frequent smaller amounts of water. Again, experience is the best teacher for learning how much water a particular plant needs on a normal watering schedule.

5. Tap a clay pot. If the plant is in a clay or ceramic pot, tap the side and listen to the sound. If you hear a dull thud, the soil is damp and the plant doesn't need more water. If you hear a higher tone, the soil is dry.

6. Use sand or gravel mixed in with the soil as a safety valve against saturation. Such additives

encourage the water to run through the soil, draining away from the roots and out the container's drainage hole.

7. Good drainage in the bottom. Improve the drainage of larger pots by keeping the holes free of roots. Place a layer of pot shards over the holes to help keep them open and the water draining freely.

8. Add perlite to your potting mix for porosity. It produces a lighter soil that won't absorb and hold as much water, although the perlite *does* hold oxygen, which is great for all those tender growing roots.

9. A number of self-watering systems are currently available that make watering easier. Although some expensive systems are designed for use in offices, public buildings, and commercial growing applications, other more affordable systems are available for home use. The main idea is to provide a water reservoir hidden in the base of the planter. Above that is a platform upon which the soil rests. A transport system allows the water to move from the reservoir to the soil above as it begins to dry out. Water is added at the same rate as it's being used up. An indicator tells when the reservoir is close to running out of water and should be refilled. The disadvantage to self-watering systems is that the soil can't be flushed out periodically of the salts that tend to build up in the soil the way it can with a normal pot, so you may have to replant in fresh soil more often.

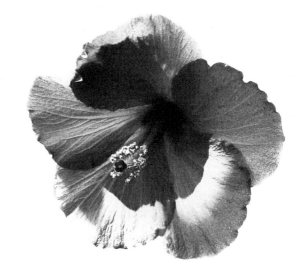

Chapter Nine:

Food for Thought

Food. The essence of life. It sustains human beings. It sustains animals. It sustains plants. To potted plants, food is especially important. Unlike those trees and shrubs growing outdoors, indoor plants receive no natural supplements to their food supply. There are no great masses of fallen leaves, no earthworm castings, no thick mats of pine needles, no nearly inexhaustible mineral deposits. Indeed, potted plants have a very exhaustible source of food: a few cubic feet of soil. Once that's gone, their only hope for sustenance is for us to come to their aid.

The very first requirements of plants are the three basics: water, air, and sunlight. Plants get water from the soil and draw carbon dioxide from the air (releasing, as a by-product of growth, the oxygen we need to sustain life). Using energy from the life-giving rays of the sun, plants combine the water and carbon dioxide

to produce a reserve of starch that they turn into sugar and use as food at night (except in a few cases) that they require in spring when growth is greatest but sunlight is still too weak to assure adequate photosynthesis.

Plants also need various mineral salts dissolved in water so their root systems can absorb them. The salts enable plants to produce fats, proteins, pigments, and other substances necessary for growth and life. These minerals include boron, copper, chlorine, iron, manganese, molybdenum, and sodium — all in tiny but critical amounts. In addition, plants require larger concentrations of nitrogen, phosphorus, and potassium.

So there's no question of whether or not indoor plants need feeding — only when, what, and how much.

There are many different ways of classifying plant food. But for simplicity's sake, we're going to divide food into two main categories: commercial and homemade. The commercial food is the stuff you buy; the home-prepared is the food you make. Neither is overwhelmingly better for your plants' health and well-being than the other; both do the job. But one may be better for your pocketbook.

Commercial Food

Commercial plant food comes in three forms: solid tablet, granulated, and liquid. The ingredients may be either synthetic (that is, chemically manufactured) or natural, such as manure, mulch, or fish emulsion. The solid and ready-to-use liquids are easier and quicker to use than the granules. Solid tablets are plugged into the soil as directed to dissolve slowly over a long period of time. The liquid is concentrated to be diluted with water before use. The granules must be mixed with water and take a little more time to break down, but they're generally less expensive.

No matter what type of commercial food you choose, it will probably be marked as to its contents. Generally, that means you'll find three numbers on the label. These numbers may be 5-5-5 or 12-18-12 or 7-3-5 — in fact, the combinations are limitless. Before buying, you should know what these numbers stand for.

The three major elements in commercial plant food are nitrogen, phosphorus, and potassium. These numbers on the plant food label correspond to the percentages of these three elements in alphabetical order. In other words, 5-5-5 means the food has 5 percent nitrogen, 5 percent phosphorus, and 5 percent potash readily available for the plants' use. The 12-18-12 formula has 12 percent nitrogen, 18 percent phosphorus, and 12 percent potash. The remainder of the food consists of various trace elements and moisture.

How does each of the three major elements contribute to a plant's health? I thought you'd never ask.

Nitrogen, often called the green-growth stimulator, is necessary for green healthy foliage. An absence of nitrogen in the soil results in leaves that look yellowish, while new leaves arrive bearing red-tinged veins.

Even though nitrogen is a plentiful substance, it's nearly always scarce in soil. That's because nitrogen is easily dissolved by water and washed away. Therefore, periodic applications of nitrogen — available in the wild from decaying vegetation — are necessary to all plants. Ammonium sulfate is the nitrogen compound most widely used in synthetic plant foods. Nitrogen is also abundant in its natural form in cottonseed meal, fish emulsions, dried blood meal, and processed sewage sludge.

Phosphorus is vital to a plant's cell production process and useful in stimulating blooms in flowering plants. When the soil lacks phosphorus, older leaves develop yellow spots, and stalks and veins become tinged with purple.

As with nitrogen, the soil rarely has enough phosphorus — especially for flowering plants. To overcome this shortage, periodic applications of phosphorus-rich food are necessary.

The forms of phosphorus most common in plant food are the mineral phosphates, for example, superphosphate. Organic sources include fish meal and bone meal.

Potash is the common name for the element potassium. It's available in most soil, and plants make good use of it. If potassium is absent, older leaves turn purple around the edges and then become reddish and brittle. Finally, the leaves crumble and fall off.

In plant foods, the most common form is potassium sulfate. As with nitrogen, watering leaches this compound out of the soil. The more you add to the soil, the more that's leached out with watering. So, it's best to add this element more regularly in several small applications rather than in one large one. Potassium sulfate is highly acidic; it's a good form of potash to use in alkaline soils because it brings the pH down toward neutral. For an already acid soil, consider using wood ashes. They contain plenty of potash, but they are alkaline and tend to reduce excess soil acidity. For fairly neutral soil, use muriate of potash, which adds potassium without changing the pH.

The next time you buy a commercial plant food, check the percentages of the three major elements carefully. If you're trying to bring a blooming tree or shrub into flower, don't use a food rich in nitrogen, such as 20-5-5. All that nitrogen will spur the growth of new greenery at the expense of the blooms. Instead, choose a food richer in phosphorus, perhaps something such as 5-20-5. That will help the plant to funnel its energy into the production of flowers and seeds.

To improve a plant's overall health and strengthen the quality and endurance of the plant, look for a food with a fairly high percentage of potash, such as 5-5-20 or 7-7-10. Remember, what you buy makes a difference in your plant's performance or growth.

One more point about commercial plant food. Some solids and granules are billed as "time-release" food. That is, you apply them as specified and they dissolve slowly, feeding the plants over a long period of time, perhaps once every 3 or 4 months. It's a terrific method of feeding plants if you hate to be bothered more than once or twice a growing season — and if you have a good memory. You shouldn't use these time-release products (or any other plant food, for that matter) more frequently than the label specifies, or you'll risk "burning out" the plants and killing them.

I have such a poor memory about such things that I'd condemn half my plants to death if I used time-release food for even 6 months. I could never remember if I fed one plant in June or April or August. Overfeeding can be very harmful to plants.

If you do manage to overfeed, there may be little you can do except sit by and watch the plant die. You may try transplanting, discarding the old soil that's drenched with food, rinsing the roots well in room-temperature water, and repotting in clean soil. Perhaps you'll be lucky, but no guarantees.

In any event, prevention is by far more effective than the cure. Be sure to follow the instructions on the label when applying any commercial plant food.

Homemade Food

The alternative to buying and using commercial plant food, of course, is using a homemade preparation. More and more indoor gardeners are leaning toward mulch and various types of mulch teas to feed their plants. These are organic materials that contain smaller percentages of the three major elements than commercial foods do. Because the organic foods have this lower concentration, they can be applied more frequently and more safely for a more uniform growing season. And they're less costly.

My favorite method of preparing indoor mulch is to collect the week's vegetable wastes, including apple cores, orange rinds, coffee grounds, and carrot and potato peelings. I place them in a blender, add a little water to facilitate things, and grind as fine as a milkshake. Then I pour the concoction into a baking tin, bake it for an hour at 350°F to evaporate some of the moisture and kill any bacteria present, and let it cool.

The next time I water, I spoon some of this mulch onto the soil and water over it. That gives the plants plenty of good, safe, nutritious food. It also aids in keeping the soil in the pot rich, loose, and full of humus.

Some indoor organic gardeners make a mulch tea to feed their plants. To give it a try, take a similar collection of vegetable wastes, tie it up in an old nylon stocking, and let the stocking hang in a quart of water, like an oversized teabag, for a few days. The result is rich in nutrients and trace elements. Boil the mixture briefly to kill off any bacteria and allow to cool before watering directly onto your plants.

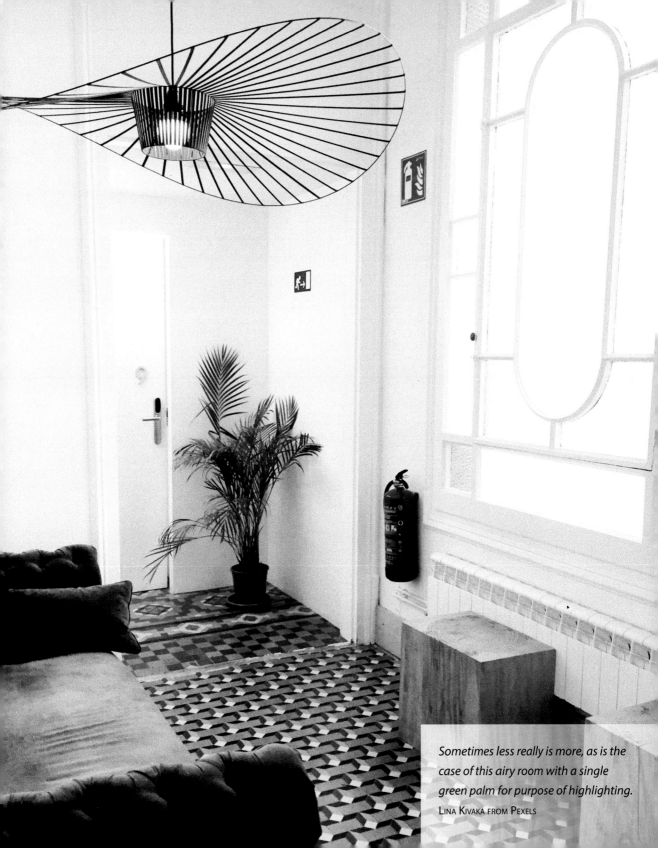

Sometimes less really is more, as is the case of this airy room with a single green palm for purpose of highlighting.

LINA KIVAKA FROM PEXELS

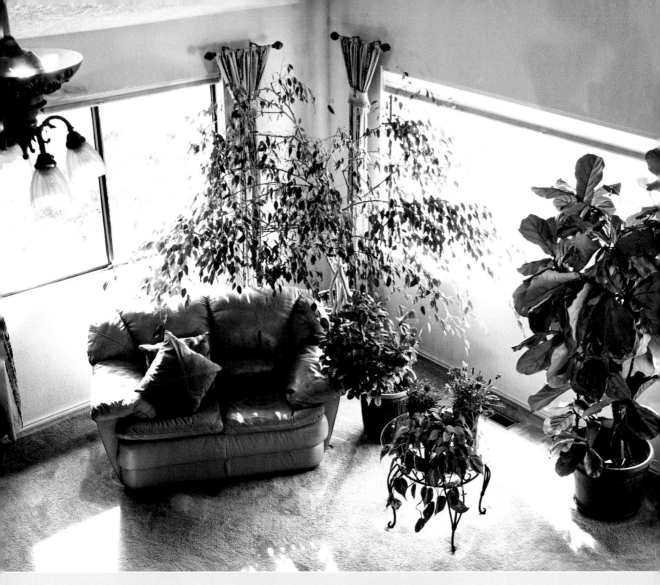

Top: *Careful placement of trees and shrubs, along with several smaller plants, can lend a warm, homey feeling to a room.* HERDA

Bottom right: *This birds-eye view shows how creative you can get when placing plants in a large room —sun-loving plants nearest the windows and shade-tolerant plants farther away.* HERDA

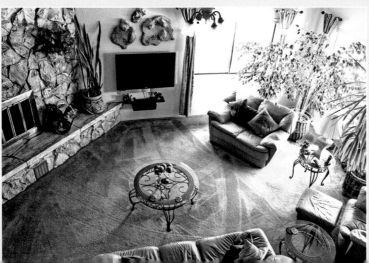

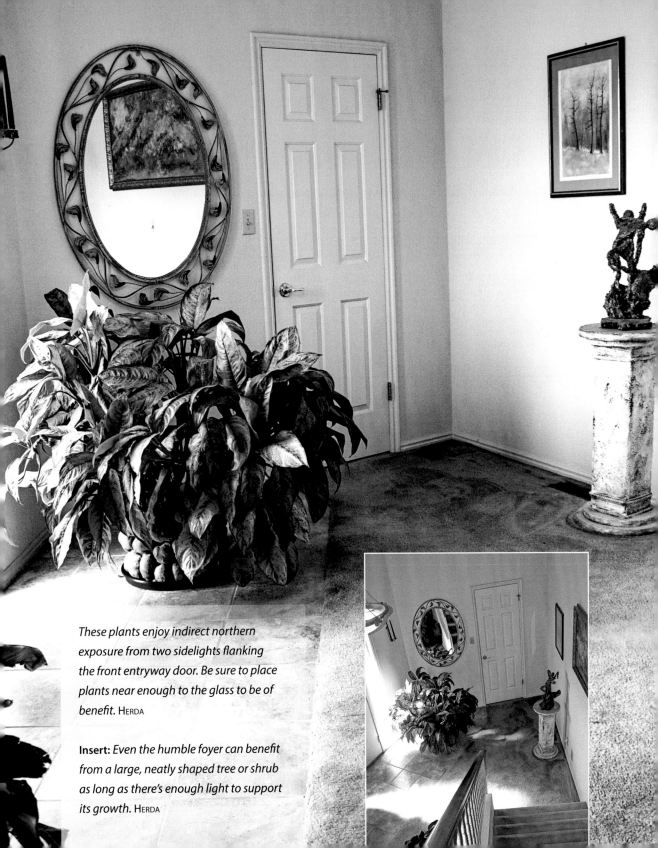

These plants enjoy indirect northern exposure from two sidelights flanking the front entryway door. Be sure to place plants near enough to the glass to be of benefit. HERDA

Insert: Even the humble foyer can benefit from a large, neatly shaped tree or shrub as long as there's enough light to support its growth. HERDA

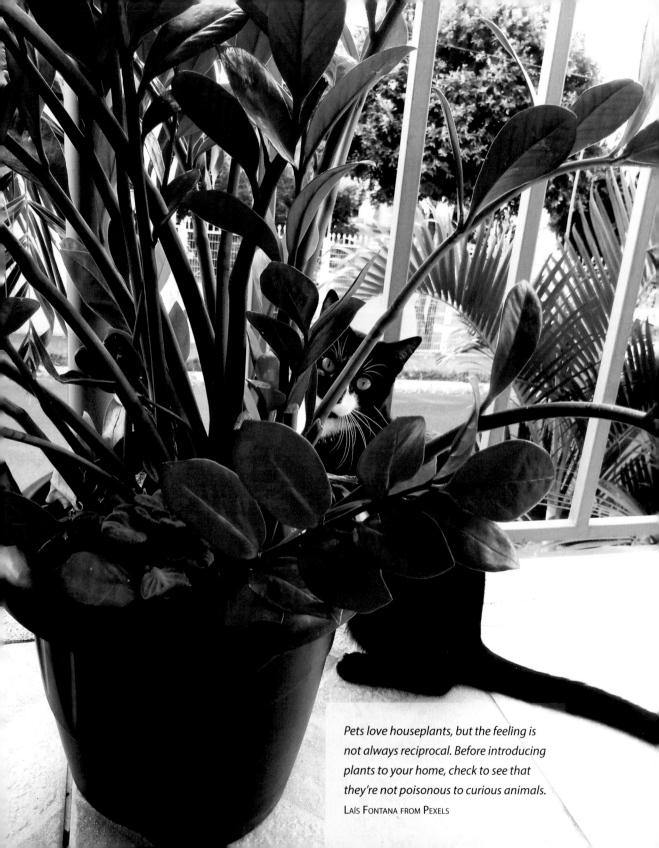

Pets love houseplants, but the feeling is not always reciprocal. Before introducing plants to your home, check to see that they're not poisonous to curious animals.

LAÍS FONTANA FROM PEXELS

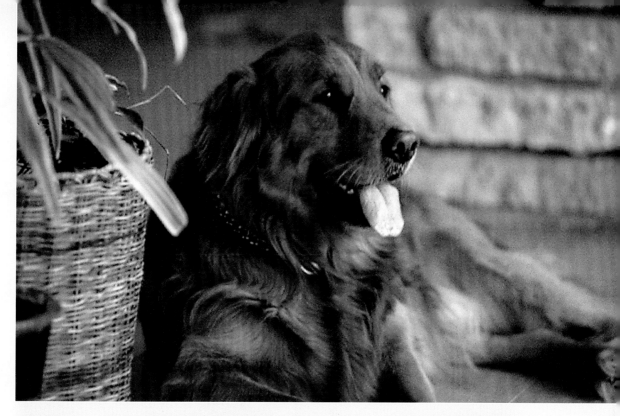

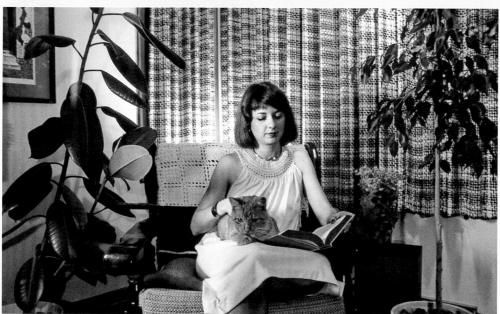

Top: *Animals often enjoy napping around healthy, hardy plants, just as they often do in the wild.* HERDA

Bottom: *A weeping fig and a rubber tree set the stage for a quiet evening at home with a good book and a sleepy kitty.* HERDA

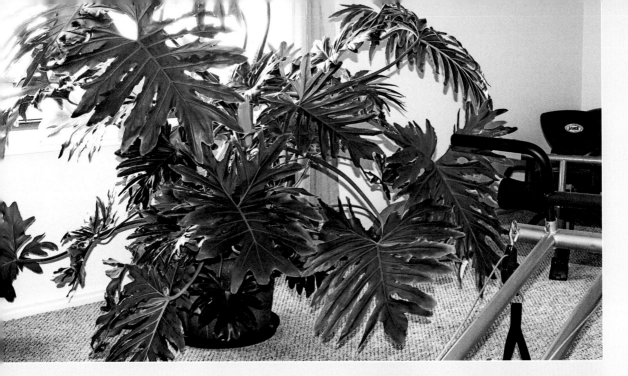

Top: *Even a crowded workout room isn't exempt from the jaw-dropping beauty of a large shrub such as this split-leaf philodendron.*
Herda

Bottom left: *Placing trees and shrubs near a light, reflective wall can help increase the amount of light your plants receive.*
Julia Kuzenkov from Pexels

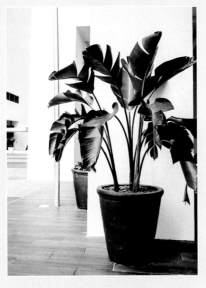

Bottom right: *A fiddleleaf fig serves as the focal point for several smaller plants and other designer elements.*
Mentatdgt from Pexels

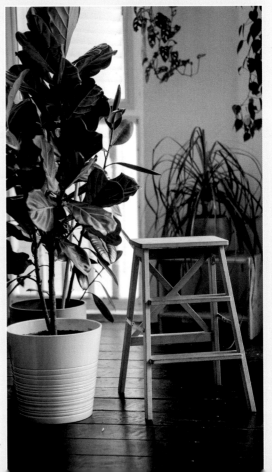

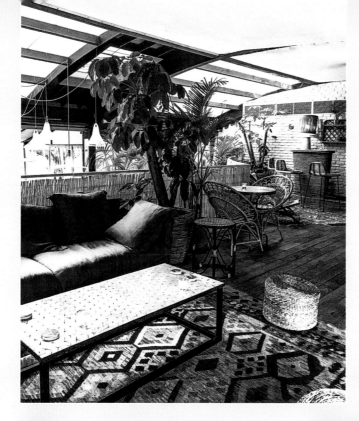

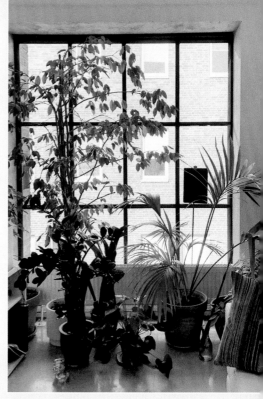

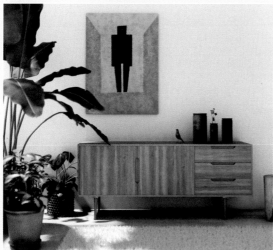

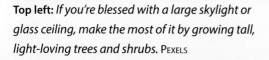

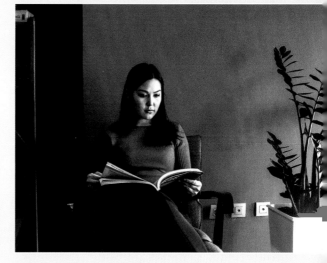

Top left: *If you're blessed with a large skylight or glass ceiling, make the most of it by growing tall, light-loving trees and shrubs.* PEXELS

Bottom left: *Grouping plants near a window rather than across the room can help keep them alive and growing vigorously.* CARLOS DIAZ FROM PEXELS

Top right: *Even a high-rise apartment can present golden opportunities for growing a wide range of plants if you have enough light.* DARIA SHEVTSOVA FROM PEXELS

Bottom right: *A single plant can often soften a colorful room, as is the case with this robust ZZ plant.* ZHANZAT MAMYTOVA FROM PEXELS

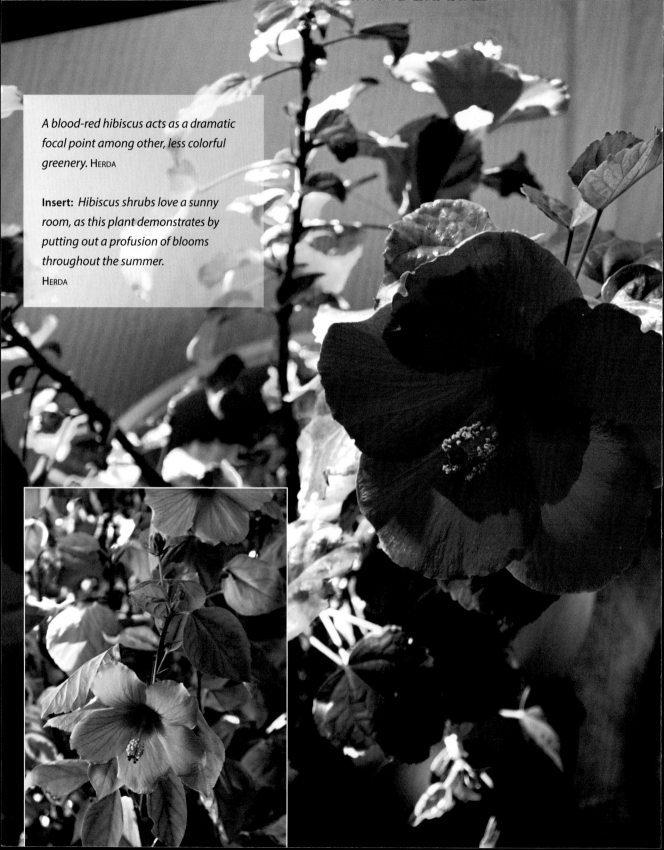

A blood-red hibiscus acts as a dramatic focal point among other, less colorful greenery. HERDA

Insert: *Hibiscus shrubs love a sunny room, as this plant demonstrates by putting out a profusion of blooms throughout the summer.*
HERDA

The tea method is fine, but if you have a lot of plants — or really large plants with plenty of soil to saturate — you're going to need several pounds of organic material steeping in five- and ten-gallon drums for the rest of your plants' lives. I'd just as soon use the grinding method.

To Feed or Not to Feed

There are times of the year when all indoor plants need feeding, and there are other times when they don't. You should generally refrain from feeding newly purchased trees or shrubs for at least 2 or 3 months. Usually, the growers who pot the plants and ship them to your local nursery or garden center have probably already applied a time-release food that will see the plants through the first several months. If you feed a newly acquired plant that has already been fed, you run the risk of double-dosing it, which could lead to trouble.

Also, avoid feeding plants during their dormant period. Deciduous trees and shrubs don't grow in fall and winter after the weather turns cold. The same is true for many evergreens. Feeding during this dormant period can trigger a plant's growth mechanism prematurely and result in spindly growth or a dangerous sapping of the plant's stored food supply.

Instead, introduce your plants to a gentle feeding program sometime in spring after you notice new growth beginning to form. Continue regular feeding until fall, when you can taper off again and stop altogether as dormancy sets in.

Science Says

Shrubs and trees require certain elements, known as macronutrients, in relatively large quantities. That's whether they're growing outside "in the wild" or indoors in a container. The most important of these elements is nitrogen (N), which is a constituent of proteins and chlorophyll that is necessary for photosynthesis and other critical plant processes.

Much of the nitrogen in potting soil is lost due to leaching out with regular watering and to volatilization (the return of nitrogen to the atmosphere as a gas). Indoor plants don't have the benefit of leaf litter and other natural sources of nitrogen, so it must be added on a regular basis. For example, raking the leaves from the lawn once each fall removes approximately 2 to 3 pounds of nitrogen for every 1,000 square feet of lawn.

Nitrogen deficiency shows up as slow growth, small leaves, and yellowing (chlorosis) foliage, especially in older leaves. On nitrogen-deficient plants, sometimes the newer, developing leaves appear greener than the older ones because nitrogen is somewhat mobile in plants, allowing it to be directed toward new growth at the expense of other parts of the plant. However, these same symptoms may also be due to other problems that affect root health and element uptake. Because nitrogen is the element most likely to be deficient in trees, fertilizer specifications usually focus on it as the most important element.

The elements phosphorous (P), potassium (K), and sulfur (S) are also necessary in fairly large amounts for healthy plant growth. These elements are often present in outdoor soil in adequate amounts for trees and shrubs, but may be leached out in containers. The secondary nutrients necessary to healthy growth include magnesium (Mg) and calcium (Ca), which are required in smaller amounts. Although these elements are called secondary, severe deficiencies can result in loss of the plant. Magnesium deficiency is an especially serious problem in palms.

Other elements, known as micronutrients, are required in lesser amounts. Still, as with the secondary elements, a deficiency of any one can have serious adverse effects on the health of the plant. Iron chlorosis, for example, is a condition that results when a tree is not absorbing sufficient quantities of iron, usually due to high soil pH (an alkaline soil). Young leaves are small and chlorotic (yellow), often with green veins, while older leaves tend to be darker green. Iron deficiency can eventually kill a tree. Like iron, manganese and zinc may at times be deficient in the soil.

The goal of fertilization is to supply nutrients that are deficient in your trees or shrubs. Trees with satisfactory growth and not showing problems of nutrient deficiency may not require fertilization. If you'd like to have your soil tested so you know for sure, contact your local nursery or arborist who can determine the exact makeup of your soil and recommend the best fertilizer for growing healthy plants.

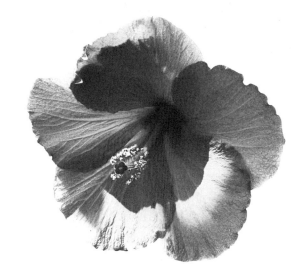

Chapter Ten:

Bugging Out!

I CAN'T THINK of a more painful experience in the life of an indoor gardener than waking up one morning to find tiny holes in the leaves of your *Ficus*. Or big, brown spots speckling your *Schefflera*. It looks like the end of a long, hard trail.

Actually, indoor gardeners are fortunate that horticultural science has advanced to a stage where there's hope and nearly a 100 percent chance for complete recovery even for plants that appear hopelessly fouled by insects or disease.

To begin with, accept the fact that your plants are going to get sick sooner or later. It's inevitable. Tiny, microscopic eggs and sometimes even the insects themselves are airborne. Each time you open a door or a window, you expose your plants to a variety of pests. Sometimes the plants' natural mechanism will successfully fight them off. Sometimes not.

Fortunately, only a few common indoor insect pests are of concern: aphids, mites, whiteflies, mealybugs, and scale. Specific insecticides, including a wide range of organic or natural products, work wonders in eliminating them without causing damage to the plants or your family. If you object to any kind of additive warfare, you can do what Suzanne, the owner of a plant shop in Chicago, does:

My *Schefflera* used to be plagued with mealybugs, scale, and spider mites, but I hated to use insecticides. Then I developed the idea of wiping the leaves with a mild solution of Ivory Liquid soap and water (never use a harsh detergent that could prove toxic to the plants). After I sponged both side of each leaf, I placed the plants in the bathtub and let the shower water rinse them clean. This also provides proper, thorough watering for the plants every 3 or 4 weeks, as necessary. Ever since I began this program, I haven't seen an insect within 20 feet of my plants.

My own evaluation of this rather unusual approach to controlling insect attack is that it's just that: control. It's not eradication. A giant *Schefflera* of mine was once attacked by spider mites. I battled them similarly by bathing each leaf and the stalks in a solution of Ivory Liquid and water. Then I tried another recommended solution, rubbing alcohol (extremely diluted) and water. After each washing, I rinsed the plant thoroughly. The only improvement I saw was that the mites seemed to be cleaner. Finally, I went to a chemical systemic followed by a potent spray. The result? I got rid of the spider mites only after getting rid of the *Schefflera*. And the insects had pretty much already taken care of that!

I don't mean to sound overly pessimistic, only realistic. I could have got rid of the spider mites and saved the *Scheff* had I used the proper approach sooner. And I believe, too, that Suzanne's approach to keeping insects from her *Schefflera* is a good one if it's practiced before serious infestation occurs. Once the bugs have grabbed control of a plant, you'll have to strike back hard and fast. But I recently added a few hidden weapons to my arsenal. More about that shortly.

Insect Pests

First, let's take a look at some of the insect pests that are most likely to show up as uninvited guests on your trees and shrubs.

Ants

Ants aren't going to be much of a problem unless your home is naturally overrun with them, or you bring them in from outdoors in the dirt balls or pots of collected specimens, or they have infested nursery-bought trees or shrubs that you bring into your home.

Ants don't damage plants directly, but they can transfer various diseases from a sick plant to a healthy one. They have the peculiar habit of picking up tiny mealybugs or aphids and moving them from place to place on host plants. Needless to say, you don't need that kind of added bug mobility. The conventional wisdom in getting rid of ants is decades old: use of a commercial ant trap — a small, enclosed tin with several holes punched in the side, containing food coated with slow-acting poison. When the ants carry the infected food back to their colony for the queen and others to feed on, poof! You can give the ants a little extra incentive by sprinkling a few grains of sugar inside the holes in the trap.

If the ants don't seem to be affected by the trap at first, have patience. These insects go through periods when they don't feed. Keep the traps around, and sooner or later they'll do the job.

Aphids

Aphids attack all parts of a plant and suck the juices from the leaves. Whole herds of these plant lice can be eradicated by hand since they can be spotted pretty easily with the naked eye. One major problem with an aphid attack is that the insects are extremely mobile. They crawl, of course, and some species fly, moving from one plant to another in a hurry if you don't take steps to isolate the infected plants. In dry, warm weather, aphids reproduce very quickly, reaching staggering numbers within a week. The young bugs mature in 2 weeks, and many are parthenogenetic (able to produce living young without fertilization); so it's easy to see how large populations can build up in a hurry.

Malathion has long been the go-to recommended insecticide. But it smells awful, and you can't help but wonder just how much damage it's doing to your own system. Although malathion is considered only mildly toxic,[1] absorption or ingestion into the human body easily results in its metabolism to malaoxon, which is substantially more toxic. Nevertheless, if you don't mind the risks, it will likely do the job. A premium grade of malathion sold as Cythion has less odor than the regular product.

Leaf Hoppers

Leaf hoppers are sometimes a problem with collected specimens. These pests tend to cling to the bottom of leaves where they're difficult to see while they eat small holes through to the surface. More damaging than that, they occasionally transmit viral diseases from sick to healthy plants. Mature adults lay eggs among a small spray of white bubbles that looks something like foamy saliva. If you notice either adults or eggs, the traditional counteractant is to spray with malathion, derris (rotenone), or BHC. Again, these chemicals have to be handled with care.

Mealybugs

Mealybugs are slow-moving insidious pests covered with a mealy wax. They look like small dabs of white cotton. But these dabs of cotton have mouths, and they like to suck the sap from a plant's leaves. They can be eradicated in small numbers by dipping a Q-Tip in alcohol and dabbing each insect lightly or by treating the plant with a liquid or crystal systemic available at most plant shops and garden centers. Mealybugs are also commonly controlled by spraying with malathion.

Mites

Mites are tiny eight-legged creatures barely visible to the unaided eye. *Spider mites*, so named because they spin tiny webs in the axils of various fleshy-leaved plants, can become serious pests: they have a short life cycle and a rapid rate of reproduction. Large populations can build up quickly under favorable conditions. You can spot them more easily by examining your plants after misting. If there are telltale webs, the droplets of water will cling to them, indicating the presence of an insect infestation. Look closely enough, and you'll actually see the white mites moving along the webs. These sucking pests are traditionally controlled with a systemic that poisons them from within the plant's veins. Until recently, Disulfoton had been the go-to systemic of choice, but Bayer abandoned the U.S. market with its product following disfavor among environmentalists. Today, spider mites are most often treated by spraying with malathion or dicofol, which is used in the production of the banned pesticide DDT. Despite concerns from environmentalists, the World Health Organization classifies dicofol as a Level II "moderately hazardous" pesticide,[2] even though it's been shown to be harmful to aquatic animals and can cause eggshell thinning in various species of birds.

Whiteflies

Whiteflies, another easily recognized pest, are small white flies (thus the name) that congregate on the underside of leaves, where they perform their dirty work. They frequently fly away when disturbed only to return almost immediately, so jostle your plants to see if they're present. They damage plants by sucking the sap, and conventional wisdom says to control them with an application of the systemic disulfoton, which has since made the Environmental Protection Agency's list of Restricted Use Products.[3] They can also be discouraged by companion planting your showpiece with African marigolds, which give off an aroma that is unpleasant to the insects.

Scales

Scales are among the most objectionable of damaging critters. They resemble small brown barnacles and attach themselves to the underside of leaves and to main stalks and shoots. These pests can best be controlled by spraying with malathion, nicotine, or a petroleum emulsion, according to conventional legend and lore.

These are the insect pests that are likely to enter your home and attack healthy plants. If you're a collector who digs up and transplants your own trees and shrubs — or if your neighbor grants you permission to transplant or even simply take cuttings to root from his property — you run a good chance of bringing still other types of insects in with you. To be on the safe side, carefully check all foliage, branches, and stems, preferably with a good, strong magnifying glass (Sherlock Holmes would have made an excellent horticulturist). If you bring in bare-root plants, check the root systems for insects or decay and, in any event, rinse the roots in a mild solution of salt water before washing clean.

If you bring in a plant with a ball of earth around the roots, pot it as soon as possible and spray the surface of the soil with an insecticide to catch any emerging insects. After that, maintain the plant in isolation for several weeks and watch for signs of trouble.

How often do you run the risk of bringing pests in with your orphan specimens? I estimate that, in my neck of the woods, two out of every three collected specimens play host to mealybug, scale, spider mites, or whitefly. Needless to say, inspection and spraying are as much a part of bringing home orphans as digging up and potting.

What to Do

The long-embraced conventional treatments for ridding your plants of insects, it's easy to see, range from the ridiculous to the outright hazardous. You may be able to rely upon the watchful eyes of Uncle Sam to protect you, but he hasn't done that great of a job so far. If you don't mind exposing your lungs and nasal passages to potential chemical carcinogens, no problem. But that's your call. Before you make it, here's what author Dave van Dallis had to say about chemical pesticides nearly fifty years ago in his article, "Safe as Directed" (*The Elks Magazine*, March 1972). It's still sound advice today.

Many chemicals marketed as pesticides over the last twenty-five years are highly toxic. Others are very persistent (long lasting) in soil, animals, and plants, building up over a period of repeated applications to absurdly high levels of toxicity. Yet all of these pesticides are for sale today on the open market with little more than a fine-print warning to alert prospective gardeners to their dangers.

"Pesticides have infiltrated our body tissues and may be ticking away like biological time bombs that could explode in the next 10 to 20 years," according to Dr. Charles S. Houston, Chairman of the Community Medicine Department at the University of Vermont. In those coming years, he added, people who will soon be producing children may store enough […] harmful pesticides in their bodies to cause serious genetic damage and birth defects to future generations. If man is able to reproduce at all.

According to Dr. Cipriano Cueto, Jr., formerly of the EPA, small quantities of pesticides were found to reduce the liver's ability to produce the enzymes controlling hormones in the body. In addition, he says, "One chemical, parathion [and its related chemical substances], accounts for some 30 to 40 deaths each year in the United States alone. That type should probably be eliminated."

With all this mind-numbing information rattling around my brain, I decided the only wise approach to using pesticides was to embark upon a fact-finding mission to locate safer alternative treatments than those mentioned above. And, you know, I found several!

Bacillus Thuringiensis

This organic pesticide is a naturally occurring bacteria that makes pests sick when they eat it. There are two strains commonly used as natural pesticides.

Bacillus thuringiensis kurstaki (Btk) gives excellent control of leaf-eating caterpillars such as cabbage worms and tomato hornworms but has no effect against insects that do not eat treated leaves. That means beneficial insects such as ladybugs and praying mantises remain unaffected! After the harmful insects eat the bacteria, their guts rupture and they die. Btk is therefore one of the safest natural pesticides for controlling caterpillar pests on vegetables or fruits without harming beneficial insects, which makes it more useful outside than indoors, where the outdoor gardener has to battle armyworms, cabbage worms, diamondback moths, melon worms, corn earworms, green cloverworms, pickleworms, tomato fruitworms, tomato hornworms, grape leafrollers, grapeleaf skeltonizers, salt marsh caterpillars, and various webworms and budworms. All are candidates for treatment with Bt.

A variance of Bt called *Bacillus thuringiensis israelensis* (Bti) can help control fungus gnats on houseplants and prevent mosquito problems in standing water in greenhouses or outdoor ponds where the water can't be drained because it contains fish.

Be aware that sunlight degrades Bt after a few hours, though, so it's best to use all of the mixture at once, preferably late in the day to be consumed during the nightly feeding frenzy. Keep in mind that your objective is to place the substance where the bugs will eat it. When using Bt to control leaf-eating pests, indoors or out, repeat treatment every 7 to 10 days until no longer needed.

Always follow label directions for diluting concentrated products of Bt and other natural pesticides. Some Bt products include genetically modified strains; products listed by the Organic Materials Review Institute (OMRI) include only naturally occurring forms.

Mix only as much Bt concentrate as you will need. If not used within a few days, dispose of unused solution by diluting it with water and pouring it out in a sunny spot to evaporate without doing any damage to the environment.

Pyrethrum

This natural insecticide made from certain species of chrysanthemum is a mixture of several different compounds called pyrethrins and cinerins. Originally pyrethrum was made by grinding dried chrysanthemum flowers into a powder. Today, it is extracted with solvents but is still widely used in household insect sprays, usually combined with another chemical called piperonyl butoxide (PBO).

Two centuries ago, people in central Asia discovered that dried, crushed flowers of certain chrysanthemums were toxic to insects. During the Napoleonic Wars (1804–1815), this "insect powder" was used to control flea and body lice infestations by French soldiers. Since then,

pyrethrum has been used in many forms for effective low-toxicity insect control. Since natural pyrethrum is not stable in sunlight, it is seldom used in commercial agriculture.

Pyrethrum insecticide, either alone or combined with other compounds, is a very safe and environmentally friendly insecticide. It is effective against a wide array of pests and can often be used even on edible crops right up to the day of harvest.

Pyrethrum is one of the botanical insecticides often combined with neem oil or insecticidal soap to make a highly effective, wide-spectrum, low-toxicity spray. These combination products can be used for aphids, scale insects, spider mites, thrips, and many other leaf-feeding pests.

Pyrethrum is a relatively low-toxicity natural insecticide, and since it breaks down quickly, it generally has low environmental impact. For these reasons, it enjoys a reputation of being "safe" for use, and it's widely available (even in many grocery stores) under various brand names. Use caution when spraying around the house, however, for it's easy to go overboard. It's not a room freshener, after all. And you have only one pair of lungs.

Diatomaceous Earth

By far, this is my favorite "new" weapon in the never-ending battle against insects. DE is composed of the fossilized remains of microscopic organisms known as *diatoms*. Their edges are sharp enough to lacerate the exoskeleton of nearly any crawling insect that comes in contact with them. Once their outer shell has been lacerated, the powdery DE dehydrates the insect, killing it (although not instantaneously). Depending upon the type of bug and other factors, you should see insects dying off in from 12 hours to 3 or 4 days.

While diatomaceous earth insecticides work well to kill most crawling insects, there are a few species that DE is known to be particularly effective against. These include ants, bedbugs, fleas, cockroaches, silverfish, most types of beetles, caterpillars, earwigs, centipedes, millipedes, sowbugs, pillbugs, spiders, crickets, and slugs.

In short, if the insect you are looking to exterminate crawls, DE will probably kill it — and absolutely safely. Apply food-grade diatomaceous earth in the cracks and crevices around your home as well as in other areas where insects are likely to enter. Leave the DE down for a few days to a week and monitor the infestation in order to judge the DE's effectiveness.

Please note: DE is likely to harm nearly any insect, including those that may be beneficial to your home or garden, so use caution when applying outdoors around ladybugs, lacewings, praying mantises, and other beneficial insects.

And one more note: Food-grade DE is not only safe for use around pets and humans (including fish), it's actually beneficial for consumption and has been credited for success when used to prevent acne and clear skin blemishes and to perform a host of other tasks.

According to Wolf Creek Ranch Animal Sanctuary:

> Some people take 1 heaping tsp. in a glass of water prior to each meal, 3x/day and swear by DE's wonderful health benefits keeping acne away, clean clear skin, better sleep, more energy, stronger hair and nails. Others take a heaping tablespoon just before bedtime … Still others put it in their protein drink, smoothies, morning coffee, etc. Whether you take DE once/day or 3x/day, everyone reports effectiveness and better health.
>
> Many women advise their hair has never been so soft as it is now since taking DE. Others advise of cleaner clear complexions, when previously they had acne trouble. Still others notice an increase in energy levels and others advise it keeps their bowels clean and helps them sleep better.... The bottom

line is it is effective in increasing our health status, as removal of internal parasites and worms will allow us to more properly absorb the nutrients from our food, as the worms/parasites will not be eating our food or sucking our blood.[4]

A word of caution: Always check with your health advisor before beginning any new personal supplemental program.

Ladies in the Parlor

As most outdoor organic gardeners can tell you, ladybugs are terrific friends to the gardener. These attractive little beetles have voracious appetites: they eat up to 200 aphids (their preferred cuisine) a day. When aphids aren't present, they'll graciously substitute mites, whitefly eggs, and even mealybugs. So what's that to you, an indoor gardener?

If destructive insects are a serious problem in your home, give some careful, unprejudiced thought to releasing from 50 to 100 ladybugs among your plants. Install a plant light above infested trees and shrubs and keep it going from dawn until dark. The light will attract the ladybugs and tend to keep them from wandering all over the house. The little beetles will stick around, gorging themselves on whatever bugs come to mandible, until their meal tickets have

been filled. Then they expire (or, if you're a softy, you can try collecting them in a butterfly net and releasing them to resume their activities outdoors).

Considering ladybugs are so inexpensive, easy to maintain (just store them dormant in the refrigerator until time for release), undemanding, and effective, you can hardly choose a better indoor insect fighter. Of course, they can't be trained to "fetch," so don't get rid of Fido.

If you like the idea of going natural but aren't sure you can tolerate even these cute little beetles congregating around the television set, move your infected plants carefully (so as not to spread the infestation around) into a hospital room such as a sunroom or spare bedroom. Release the ladybugs, and close the door. Once they've done the job, just open a window, and they'll be gone within a day.

Ladybugs are available by mail from several sources or from your local garden center or nursery.

Insecticidal Soap

The active ingredient in insecticidal soap comes from the fatty acids in animal fat or vegetable oil, so it's important to use an organic soap such as Dr. Bronner's Pure Castile Soap or other brands readily available online and in most grocery stores. Do not use detergents (which aren't really soap), dish soaps, or any other products containing degreasers, skin moisturizers, or synthetic chemicals, or you'll risk killing your plants. To make a 2% insecticidal soap solution (the most common dilution), combine 5 tablespoons of pure liquid soap with 1 gallon of water or 1 heaping tablespoon of soap to 1 quart of water. Spray as required to saturate the tops and undersides of leaves, stems, and soil surface. Repeat as required.

Plant Diseases

Plant diseases are another, although less frequent, scourge of indoor gardeners that require a different approach than those above. The diseases are caused by fungi, bacteria, or viruses and include several groups: soil-dwelling fungi, branch fungi, gray molds, rust fungi, leaf spot fungi, and mildew. Among the most commonly encountered bacterial diseases are rot, leaf spot, and gall.

There are a number of effective treatments for various plant diseases, whether fungal, bacterial, or viral. The various symptoms and cures are far too complex a subject for coverage in a book of this scope. To cope with them, you may need help from an expert in the field.

If your trees and shrubs come under attack from something that you suspect is a disease rather than an insect, turn to the sage advice of your local horticulturist or county agent or, if that's not possible, to your garden-center specialist. If you fail to find someone willing or able to come to your rescue, the burden is on you. Jump on the Internet, do a search for the symptoms plaguing your plant, and take the best advice you find. Or go to your local library or bookstore and pick up a copy of *Garden Pests and Diseases of Flowers and Shrubs,* by Mogens Dahl and Thyge B. Thygesen, or *Plant Disease Handbook,* by Cynthia Westcott. They're two of the better books I've found on the subject.

Short of that, the following primer on plant diseases may prove useful.

Some 85 percent of plant diseases are caused by fungal or fungal-like organisms, although other serious diseases can be caused by viral or bacterial organisms. Nematodes, too, can cause plant disease. Other diseases, called noninfectious "abiotic" diseases, result from air pollution, nutritional deficiencies, or toxicities that result in less than desirable growth, according to research conducted by the Michigan State University Agricultural Extension.

If plant disease is suspected, careful attention to the appearance of the plant can offer a good clue as to the type of pathogen involved.

A **sign of plant disease** is physical evidence of the pathogen. For example, fungal fruiting bodies are a sign of disease. When you look at powdery mildew on a lilac leaf, you're actually looking at the parasitic fungal disease organism itself (*Microsphaera alni*). Bacterial canker of stone fruits causes gummosis, a bacterial exudate, or a substance that oozes out from plant pores, emerging from the cankers. The thick liquid exudate is primarily composed of bacteria and is a sign of the disease, although the canker itself is composed of plant tissue and is a symptom.

A **symptom of plant disease** is a visible effect of disease on the plant. Symptoms may include a detectable change in color, shape, or function of the plant under attack by the pathogen. Leaf wilting is a typical symptom of verticilium wilt, caused by the fungal plant pathogens, *Verticillium albo-atrum* and *V. dahliae*. Common bacterial blight symptoms include brown necrotic lesions surrounded by a bright yellow halo at the leaf margin or interior of the leaf on certain plants. You are not actually seeing the disease pathogen itself, but rather a symptom that is caused by the pathogen.[5]

Here are a few examples of common signs and symptoms of fungal, bacterial, and viral plant diseases:

Fungal disease signs:
- Leaf rust (common leaf rust in corn)
- Stem rust (wheat stem rust)
- Sclerotinia (white mold)
- Powdery mildew

Fungal disease symptoms:
- Birds-eye spot on berries (anthracnose)
- Damping off of seedlings (phytophthora)
- Leaf spot (septoria brown spot)
- Chlorosis (yellowing of leaves)

Bacterial disease signs (difficult to observe, but can include):
- Bacterial ooze
- Water-soaked lesions
- Bacterial streaming in water from a cut stem

Bacterial disease symptoms:
- Leaf spot with yellow halo
- Fruit spot
- Canker
- Crown gall
- Shepard's crook stem ends on woody plants

Viral disease signs:
- None (the viruses themselves can't be seen)

Viral disease symptoms:
- Mosaic leaf pattern
- Crinkled leaves
- Yellowed leaves
- Plant stunting

You can see that there is a lot of overlap between fungal, bacterial, and viral disease symptoms. Also, abiotic diseases, herbicide injury, and nematode problems must be considered possibilities when an unknown plant problem appears. This list is not complete but rather an example of some of the more common diseases.

What to Do

Once you identify the type of pathogen attacking your plant, either through personal observation or with the aid of an expert, you'll need to make a quick trip to your favorite nursery or horticultural supply center. There you'll find plenty of different products — fungal, bacterial, and viral — along with someone to offer advice on how best to use each one. Pay attention to any safe-handling warnings on the label, and always be sure to dispose of leftover fungicides as if they were hazardous materials, which some may be.

Also, whenever possible, try moving your infected plants to a hospital room — a room that can be shut off from the rest of the house — so that you can treat all the plants at once and prevent the disease from spreading to your healthy plants.

Insecticides, Pesticides, and Pathogenicides

Assuming your plants are free of disease but still vulnerable to insect attack, the question always arises: What would you use, an organic or inorganic insecticide? That merits more than a little consideration.

Commercial inorganic insecticides are quick, precise, and targeted. They're also dangerous as hell. The question then becomes this: Is it worth the risk?

I consider myself an organic gardener. I mulch my outdoor vegetable garden and wouldn't come within 50 feet of it with an inorganic insecticide. But, outdoors, I don't have to. When insects strike, as they do every year, there are always natural checks around to draw upon. There are ladybugs and praying mantises to release in the garden. There are birds to attract to feast on the pests. There are harmless powders (such as finely screened lime and that miracle of all pesticides, diatomaceous earth) to sprinkle over plants to keep harmful insects away. There are pest-repellent flowers to plant and traps to set. Together, these stratagems work well enough to assure that I'm left with a majority of the crop by the end of the season. And that's good enough for me.

But indoors is another matter. There, I use organic insect control wherever possible. And since I've been doing that, I haven't gone near an inorganic commercial insecticide, let alone purchased one, in more than 10 years.

But, where fungal, bacterial, and viral disease pathogens are concerned, I recognize that, sooner or later, I'm going to have to buy the best product to do the job and that it may have to be inorganic. But which product? It does make a difference.

Before World War II, we knew preciously little about chemical warfare. Afterwards, we knew plenty. An explosion of pest-control research that began in the 1940s provided a steady stream of data and many "new" compounds effective against an army of destructive insects. Lead arsenate, Paris Green, and hellebore had once been the common garden insecticides, but postwar gardeners found the chlorinated hydrocarbons, such as DDT, chlordane, dieldrin, and the organic phosphates, more effective. Over the last half century and more, these compounds have been not only used but abused … badly.

One avenue of research concerns ways of sterilizing insects so that they are unable to reproduce in quantities large enough to do serious damage. Some kinds of insects have been sterilized by radiation and others have had their reproductive capacity altered chemically. While sterilization by radiation is certainly not a home remedy, it does illustrate the wide range of practices employable in stopping destructive insects dead in their tracks. But you shouldn't try to kill an elephant with a fly swatter, nor should you use a Sherman tank to smash an ant! The key to successful and effective use of any

insecticide is to match the method to the problem.

So far as battling insects goes, many types of insecticides are available to the indoor gardener. They include inorganic chemicals, microbial insecticides, botanical insecticides, chlorinated hydrocarbons, organic phosphates, systemic insecticides, carbamates, oil sprays, miticides, and poison baits. For various reasons, some are less suitable than others to use indoors. Those that I recommend, when called for, include these:

Botanical Insecticides. As the name implies, these are insecticides obtained from crushed or powdered parts of plants. They're safe for humans and most wildlife. This group includes nicotine for fighting aphids and various other sucking insects; pyretheum for sucking insects and flies; rotenone, a general insecticide (it's harmful to fish, so avoid use near indoor pools and aquariums); and sabadilla, a general insecticide with less killing power than rotenone.

Organic Phosphates. These insecticides kill by disabling the nervous system. They may be used with caution outdoors, on the porch, or in the garage, but some products in this group should not be used indoors. Be especially careful to read the labels on these products before purchase and use. Malathion, the most widely used organic phosphate, kills scales, whiteflies, mealybugs, and other insects. Diazinon, which is marketed under the name Spectracide, is a general broad-range insecticide. TEPP, for aphids, mites, and other sucking insects, is highly toxic to humans, but its toxicity breaks down quickly.

Systemic Insecticides. These chemicals are absorbed through the roots of plants and distributed throughout the plants' systems. Sucking insects and mites that feed on the treated plants are poisoned. Although not recommended for food crops, for obvious reasons, systemics (especially the powders and granules) are generally safe, effective means of dealing with sucking pests in indoor and outdoor plants. Do not use where dirt-eating pets or young children are present! Included in this group are bidrin, demeton (under the name Systox), phosdrin, and phorate (under the name Thimet).

Miticides. As the name implies, these insecticides are formulated expressly for control of mites. Perhaps the most widely used indoors is dicofol (under the name Kelthane). Others include ovex (under the name Ovotran), aramite, and dimite. The last two are not to be used on food crops.

Dormant Oil Sprays. This group includes various emulsified oils for the control of scale insects, mealybugs, and the eggs of many insects and mites. The sprays are used on dormant trees. Oil sprays may injure thin-barked trees such as beech, birch, hickory, and maple and should be used on these trees only as a last resort. A good example is oil dormant (under the name Superior Oil); best used on plants that overwinter outdoors.

Summer Oil Sprays. These insecticides are used for certain insect infestations during the plants' active growing season. They have characteristics similar to those of dormant oil sprays. A good example is oil summer (under the name Superior Oil). It's especially effective for fighting mites and scale on citrus trees when everything else has failed.

Diatomaceous Earth. Finally, if it crawls, clings, sucks, flies, swarms, or otherwise maneuvers itself into position to attack your plants, it's susceptible to DE. Diatomaceous earth is a natural mineral that is so fine, it physically penetrates the tough exoskeleton of numerous troublesome insects, thus exposing their systems to dehydration and death. It works on everything from mites and whitefly to ants and roaches. As a bonus, it's absolutely harmless to fish, birds, amphibians, and primates (including you and me). In fact, DE is beneficial to the human diet since it's so rich in minerals. It's often found in many foodstuffs we consume.

Will it work on fungus, bacteria, and other similar plant diseases? No insecticide will. But continuing scientific exploration of fungal diseases in particular is also generating new knowledge in biological methods of controlling and eradicating fungal plant pathogens.

Science Says

Pathogen-caused leaf spot diseases, particularly those of stone fruit trees and vegetables such as tomato, pepper, and lettuce, are of two types: those caused by bacteria, and those caused by fungus. They are generally similar in appearance and effect and often require the same prevention and treatment practices.

Fungal and Bacterial Leaf Spot

Plants infected with either fungal or bacterial leaf spot have water-spot type markings on the foliage, sometimes with a yellow halo and usually uniform in size. The spots enlarge and will run together under wet conditions. Under dry conditions, the spots have a speckled appearance. As spots become more numerous, entire leaves may yellow, wither, and drop.

Fungal leaf spot attacks ornamental and food crops. **Bacterial leaf spot** will additionally infect some annual and perennial flowering plants such as geraniums, zinnias, purple coneflowers, and black-eyed Susan, as well as aspen and poplar trees. Leaf spot can also cause problems for strawberry plants.

Both types of leaf spot are most active when there is plenty of moisture and warm temperatures. During the summer months, especially if plants are watered by overhead sprinklers, sufficient moisture may be present for infection when the bacteria are splashed around or blown onto leaves.

This disease overwinters in the soil around infected plants as well as on garden debris and seeds. It will also remain in the twig cankers, leaves, stems, and fruit of infected trees.

Control

Indoors, provide adequate air circulation for your plants, and disinfect your pruning equipment (1 part bleach to 4 parts water) after each cut. There is no cure for plants infected with bacterial leaf spot, but you can help prevent it through the following techniques:

- Spraying with a baking soda solution (1 tablespoon of baking soda, 2½ tablespoons of vegetable oil, and 1 teaspoon of liquid soap — not harsh detergent — in 1 gallon of water.) Spraying with neem oil may also help. Spray only a few leaves and check for negative reactions before applying every 2 weeks.

• Apply sulfur sprays or copper-based fungicides weekly at first sign of disease to prevent its spread. These organic fungicides will not kill leaf spot but will prevent the spores from germinating.[6]

Fungal Infections

Diseases caused by fungal pathogens take their energy from the plants on which they live. They are responsible for a great deal of damage, both residentially and commercially, characterized by wilting, scabs, moldy coatings, rusts, blotches, and rotted tissue.[7] Annual estimated losses to food crops alone exceed 40 percent worldwide.

Until recently, the only tools a home gardener had against fungal diseases were inorganic chemical compounds, with several exceptions. Copper, neem oil, and even everyday baking soda have been used as fungicides with some degree of success for decades. Today, however, numerous commercially organic fungicides are available. Although safer in application than their older, more established inorganic chemical counterparts, care must still be utilized in handling these organic compounds and substances. While they are safer to use around people and animals than inorganic

compounds, some products can cause health issues if misused or mishandled. Always read the warnings and instructions of any new product before use.

Here are some commonly available commercial fungal products that rely upon organic ingredients to kill a wide range of harmful pathogens, insects, or both.

Monterey Bi-Carb for powdery mildew. Active ingredients: micro-encapsulated potassium bicarbonate (baking soda). Description: A contact fungicide, it disrupts the potassium ion balance in the fungus cell causing the cell walls to collapse. Use on roses, vegetables, grapes, fruit trees, and ornamentals.

Safer Brand 3-in-1 Garden Spray for powdery mildew, black spot, leaf spot, rust, aphids, leaf-feeding caterpillars, crickets, earwigs, lace bugs, leafhoppers, mealybugs, mites, plant bugs, immature scale, thrips, and whiteflies. Active ingredients: Potassium salts of fatty acids (soap) and sulfur. Description: Provides three garden solutions in one: fungicide, insecticide, and miticide. Kills pests and creates an environment where damaging fungi cannot live. Can be applied directly to fruits and vegetables right up to the day before harvest.

Monterey 70% Organic Neem Oil for black spot, powdery mildew, rusts, scabs, whiteflies, aphids, and scales. Active ingredients: Clarified hydrophobic extract of neem oil. Description: A broad-spectrum insecticide, miticide, and fungicide, this controls numerous diseases as well as insects and mites. Use on vegetables, fruit trees, ornamentals and more, up to day of harvest. Kills eggs, larvae, and adult insects. Use indoors or out on trees, shrubs, flowering plants, fruits, and vegetables.

Actinovate Lawn and Garden for root rot, damping off, turf brown patch, club root, grey snow mold, pink snow mold, foliar diseases, powdery mildew, downy mildew, grey mold, black spot, leaf spots, rusts, fire blight, walnut blight, bacterial spot, citrus canker, bacterial blast, and peach leaf curl. Active ingredients: *Streptomyces lydicus*. Description: A one-stop fungus fighter for gardens, lawns, and hydroponics. Actinovate works from root to leaf with a concentrated beneficial microorganism (*Streptomyces lydicus*) that establishes itself on plants' roots and leaves. This water-soluble organic fungicide knocks back diseases that attack your lawn, ornamentals, and even edibles, yet is proven to be safe around pets, people, and the environment.

Bonide Garden Dust for pine needle blight, powdery mildew, black spot, rusts, ants, aphids, beetles, moths, leafhoppers, whiteflies, mites, stink bugs, and web worms. Active ingredients: Pyrethrins, sulfur, and copper. Description: Bonide Garden Dust is specially formulated to control both insect pests and plant diseases. May be applied as a spray or dust on most vegetables, fruits, and flowers. Contains a powerful blend of pyrethrins, sulfur, and copper. Colored green to blend with foliage.

Mycostop Biological Fungicide for pythium, fusarium, botrytis, alternaria, phomopsis, rhizoctonia, wilt, root rot, and phytophthora. Active ingredients: Dried spores and mycelium of *Streptomyces griseoviridis*. Description: Developed from a naturally occurring bacteria, *Streptomyces griseoviridis*, Mycostop Biological Fungicide thrives in the root zone of plants. When applied as a drench or spray, the dried spores and mycelium of the *Streptomyces* culture germinate and begin to grow on and around the plant's roots. In doing so, they create a biological defense against root-infecting pathogenic fungi that cause disease such as wilt and root rot. Mycostop has been shown to increase plant vigor and yields, even in the absence of obvious root pathogen activity. The explanation is that the *Streptomyces* produce root-stimulating hormones (demonstrated in the lab), while the *Streptomyces* control minor root pathogens that slowly feed on and damage roots.[8]

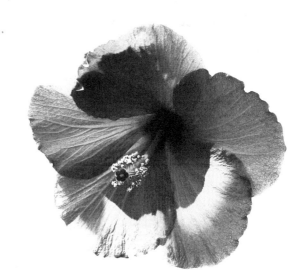

Chapter Eleven:

Propagating Your Indoor Plants

WHEN I WAS YOUNG, I considered propagation a strange and formidable-sounding concept, one that nice people didn't talk about in mixed company. Occasionally, though, I'd drop some seeds into the earth or take a cutting, stick it in some moist sand, and wait to see what happened.

The years went by, and my houseplant collection expanded from a couple of *Coleus* and *Philodendron* to include *Dracaena, Ficus, Acer* (maples), *Malus* (apples), *Pinus* (pines), *Thuja* (arborvitae), and more. In the process, my understanding of propagation expanded too. Today, I think of propagating as something more than a way to kill a rainy afternoon; I think of it as an absolute necessity.

A catalog from my local nursery has prices not too much higher or lower than those advertised by nurseries everywhere. It shows such plants as *Althea, Buddleia,*

dogwood, *Cotoneaster, Forsythia,* honeysuckle, *Magnolia*, birch, and locust, ranging from under $5 to more than $30. And the exotic plants run even higher! You get the picture. If I had to buy each plant I set my heart upon bringing home, I'd still be at the *Coleus* and *Philodendron* stage of my life. For me, propagating is a necessity. And the wondrous part of it is — it's easy.

Montague Free, in his *Plant Propagation in Pictures*, lists several categories of propagation.[1] These include propagation by seeds and spores; asexual division; stem cuttings; bulbs, corms, tubers, rhizomes, and rootstocks; runners, offsets, stolons, and suckers; layering; and grafting. For our purposes in dealing with trees and shrubs, we'll discuss the four most common forms of propagation: seeds; root division; air layering; and softwood and hardwood cuttings.

Of these four categories, one — propagation by seed — is sexual; the others are asexual or vegetative (involving propagation by the plant's own vegetation). I've settled on these four because, in my opinion, they're the ones you're most likely to use. If you'd like additional information on propagating, I highly recommend Free's book, as well as *Wyman's Gardening Encyclopedia* by Donald Wyman, a classic reference for the serious indoor or outdoor gardener.

Seeds

Growing plants from seeds is one of the most basic and simplest methods of propagating, although not necessarily always best. For the most hassle-free experience, purchase your seeds from a reliable source, follow planting instructions, and wait for the magic to happen.

If you want a plant whose seeds are not available to purchase or simply would like to harvest your own, the "simple" part of the process gets a little more involved. For starters, collecting seeds from some species of indoor trees and shrubs can be difficult because the parent plants may refuse to flower and seed under typical indoor growing conditions. Or, if they do, they may not develop fertile seeds unless conditions are just right. Even if your indoor plants flower and develop fertile seeds, they may not germinate readily. For such stubborn plants, other means of propagation are best.

Although more flowering plants are produced from seed than any other means, some plants do not produce offspring true to their varieties from seed. To understand why, think of a seed as a plant's means of sexually reproducing itself. As in human beings, an embryo from a seed may have many of its parents' characteristics, but it's an entirely new and different individual and never an exact duplicate of its parents. Some plants do produce offspring true to their species; others, particularly varietal hybrids, do so only in rare instances.

Seeds from hybrids may produce offspring that are far more spindly than their parents, for example. The plantlets may lack the unusual coloring that attracted you to a certain hybrid variety in the first place. They may lack the disease resistance of the parent plants or be unable to grow under as wide a range of conditions. As a result, the young plantlet produced from hybrid seed may be practically worthless. Nobody wants to plant corn and get stinging nettle!

On the bright side, most non-hybridized trees and shrubs do produce offspring true to their variety from seed. To enable you to know which is which, I've indicated some of those species and varieties that do not produce well from seed in the listings later in the book.

Not All Seeds Are Alike

Some seeds need special preparation before planting. For example, the seeds of apple trees and other fruit trees have fleshy coverings, as do the seeds of the barberry, *Cotoneaster,* dogwood, *Moringa,* and holly. In such cases, you should remove the covering before sowing. In general, seeds with a hard coating should be soaked in a pan of room-temperature water overnight to speed germination. Seeds with a soft covering need not be soaked.

For best success, sow seeds in a flat or a small pot of soil consisting of about one-third peat moss, one-third sterile garden soil, and one-third compost. Cover the seeds with fine sterilized soil to a depth equal to twice the diameter of the seed (i.e., not very deep!) and keep moist but not saturated. Or you may choose to sow your seeds in one of the many commercial seeding mixtures or in peat pellets that expand to pot-sized mounds when water is added.

Some trees, like maple, willow, and poplar, ripen their seeds early in the year; their seeds are usually short-lived. Such seeds must be sown as soon as they ripen because they'll lose their vitality if allowed to dry out.

Those trees and shrubs that have relatively large seeds, including ash, oak, linden, and Euonymus, can be planted as soon as the seed is ripe and detached from the parent plant. Other seeds may be sowed when ripe, or they may be stored. If such seeds are kept in dry, airtight containers, they will still germinate a year or more after ripening. These include the smaller seeds of hemlock, spruce, fir, larch, and other conifers, as well as those of *Philadelphus* (mock orange) and *Spiraea.* Other seeds in this category include Alnus, Azalea, *Betula, Buddleia, Catalpa, Clethra, Deutzia, Diervilla, Erica, Evodia, Hydrangea, Hypericum, Kalmia, Kolkwitzia, Phellodendron,* and *Thuja.* The plants whose seeds can be dried and stored before sowing are described later in the book.

Some seeds of woody plants require a dormant period before they'll germinate. Single dormant seeds need a period of cold temperature before planting. Double dormant seeds require a period of warm temperature followed by a second period of cold temperature before sowing. In the wilds, this double dormancy lasts for a year or two, depending on the type of seed. But by a simple procedure known as *stratification,* you can speed up the period of dormancy dramatically.

Single Dormancy Seeds

The plants listed below are those whose seeds are single dormant. To propagate these, collect the seeds and clean away any pulpy or fleshy covering. Allow the seeds to air-dry for a day or two. Then proceed with the mixing and storing process called stratification.

First, fill a polyethylene bag with a mixture of half sand and half peat moss. Moisten the mixture and work in the seeds so that they're stratified throughout the soil. To be sure you know how long to store them, mark the removal date on the bag with a felt-tip pen or waterproof grease marker. For example, single dormant seeds bagged on January 1 should be marked for removal sometime between February 1 and May 1, depending on the recommended stratification time listed in the chart below.

The last step is to place the bag of seeds in cold storage of about 40°F for 1 to 4 months, depending on the variety. As luck would have it, the average refrigerator temperature is around 40°F. Place the bag in an unused corner of the refrigerator (not in the freezer compartment) and check from time to time for signs of sprouting, or germination.

Here's a list of single-dormancy trees and shrubs and their stratification time at 40°F:

- *Acer* (maple), 3 mos.
- *Berberis* (barberry), 3 mos.
- *Betula* (birch), 2 to 3 mos.
- *Cornus florida* (flowering dogwood), 3 mos.
- *Fagus* (beech), 3 mos.
- *Fraxinus* (ash), 2 to 3 mos.
- *Ligustrum* (privet), 3 mos.
- *Magnolia*, 1 mo.
- *Malus* (apple), 1 to 2 mos.
- *Pinus*, 2 mos.
- Prunus (cherry, plum, etc.), 3 to 4 mos.
- *Thuja* (arborvitae), 2 mos.

Double Dormancy Seeds

Certain plants, including *Cotoneaster, Davidia, Ilex, Juniperus, Taxus,* and *Viburnum,* may take up to 2 years to germinate in the wild. Stratification is especially valuable in reducing the double-dormancy period of these plants.

First, collect and clean the seeds and stratify them with soil in a plastic bag, as in single dormancy procedures. Tie the bag tightly, and label it with two removal dates (warm and cold). It should stay in a warm place (65° to 85°F) for 4 to 6 months before being moved to the refrigerator at about 40°F for 3 months. Double dormant seeds include *Cotoneaster, Crataegus, Davidia, Ilex, Juniperus, Rhus, Taxus,* and *Viburnum.*

After stratification of either single dormant or double dormant seeds has been completed, the stratified soil mass may be removed from the bag by splitting the plastic along the side. Plant the entire mass in a large pot and cover with a clear plastic bag or a piece of glass to help retain soil moisture. Keep the soil moist as the young seedlings emerge, but don't saturate the soil or you'll drown the delicate young plants.

Poke a few holes in the plastic bag or tilt up the glass for a while each day to permit air circulation and to discourage the formation of fungus and mold. Give the seedlings good light but not strong sunlight. (You don't want to cook them, remember.) When the seedlings have developed two or three sets of "true" leaves, they may be transplanted to individual pots.

The following list of trees and shrubs indicates which seeds may be sown as soon as ripe (r), which must be stratified (s), and which may be stored dry (d) and sown at any time within the period of a year.

No seed, of course, will germinate unless it's ripe. But how do you know if a particular seed is ripe? That's an interesting question. The ripening dates vary not only from one genus to another but also among species within the same genus, so no generalization will hold true. One of the best ways to collect seeds that may be stored or stratified after ripening is to wait until the tree or shrub sheds them naturally. For those seeds that should be sown immediately upon ripening though, it's best to obtain a list of the ripening dates, or collection dates, known for native North American plants. Such a list should be available from your county agent or horticultural extension agency or by writing the Arnold Arboretum in Boston, Massachusetts.

Root Division

Another means commonly used for plant propagation is root division, one

- *Acer* (r)
- *Actinidia* (d)
- *Berberis* (s)
- *Betula* (s)
- *Buxus* (s)
- *Cedrus* (r)
- *Cornus* (s)
- *Cotoneaster* (s)
- *Fagus* (r)
- *Franklinia* (r)
- *Fraxinus* (d)
- *Hibiscus* (d)
- *Juniperus* (s)
- *Laburnam* (d)
- *Lagerstroemia* (d)
- *Ligustrum* (s)
- *Magnolia* (r)
- *Mahonia* (r)
- *Malus* (s)
- *Phellodendron* (s)
- *Philadelphus* (d)
- *Pinus* (d)
- *Prunus* (s)
- *Salix* (r)
- *Thuja* (d)
- *Viburnum* (s)
- *Zelkova* (r)

of the oldest and simplest methods. It involves cutting the stalks and roots of an existing plant apart with a spade knife or pulling them apart after the plant has been unearthed, in other words, dividing it. Shrubs such as *Spiraea*, mock orange, honeysuckle, and false *Spirea*, among others, adapt well to division. The most important thing to remember about division is when to practice it. For the most success, do it while the plant is dormant, in either early spring (for late-blooming plants) or late fall (for early-blooming plants).

Make sure each newly divided clump has an adequate root mass to support its above-ground growth. After dividing and transplanting, keep the plant out of direct sunlight until new root growth has a chance to take place. Even if the plant normally prefers direct light, give it good indirect light for 1 month or so before gradually introducing it to full sun.

Air Layering

This is perhaps the most involved and least practiced form of propagation, although it's by no means difficult to accomplish. It involves scarifying, or injuring, the stem of a woody plant, inserting an object into the wound, wrapping moist peat moss around the area, and keeping the moss damp until rooting occurs. It's an excellent way to cut back an old plant that has grown too tall for its indoor surroundings and, at the same time, produce a new plant with the identical characteristics of the old one.

To illustrate, let's assume you have a 6-foot-tall rubber plant that you'd like to cut back to 4 feet. You'd also like another rubber plant for your efforts. Four feet above the plant's base, gash the stem with a vertical slit about 2 inches long. Stuff a small twig or a hard wad of moss into the slit to prevent it from sealing itself closed. (The plant's natural tendency is to heal the "wound.")

Next, dust the wound with a root-inducing hormone such as Rootone™, Click Clone, Take Root, etc. Wrap a fist-sized ball of dampened moss around the stem so that it covers the slit and extends a couple of inches above and below the wound. Finally, seal the entire ball of moss with plastic wrap to conserve moisture. Tie the top and bottom of the plastic securely against the stem with twist ties or twine so that no air can enter. If the plant is in a sunny location, cover the wrap with aluminum foil or some other material to prevent sun scald.

If you've carefully sealed off the plastic film so the moss won't dry out, you'll notice roots showing through the moss within a couple of months. (Sorry, I never said this was a quick process.) When the roots are well developed, remove the plastic wrap, sever the stem below the rooted mass, and plant the newly rooted plantlet. It should soon develop new branches. You'll end up with your original rubber plant (now 4 feet tall), which should send out multiple new stalks from the cut, plus a well-rooted 2-foot-tall youngster with identical traits to the parent plant.

The success of air layering depends upon the time of year it's practiced, the size of the stem or branch that is cut, the amount of hormone powder dusted on, and the moisture content maintained in the moss. Remember that, since the polyethylene allows next to no moisture to escape, the moss shouldn't be saturated, only damp. It's a good practice to soak the moss thoroughly and then squeeze out all the excess moisture before entombing it in plastic. For most species, the best time to practice air layering is early spring on wood that's dormant, or in midsummer on that year's new growth.

What's the main drawback to air layering? In tests conducted at the Arnold Arboretum, the method proved to be effective about 50 percent of the time. That means it failed about 50 percent of the time, not a very heart-warming figure, admittedly. (I doubt that Jimmy the Greek would make book on it.) Still, the technique of air layering is so practical that it's definitely worth trying on plants that have grown too tall for their surroundings.

Some of the plants that responded successfully to air layering in a series of experiments at the Arnold Arboretum include these:

- *Acer* (several species)
- *Betula* (several species)
- *Corylus chinensis*
- *Cotoneaster foveolata; C. horizontalis*
- *Davidia involucrata vilmorinii*
- *Hibiscus syriacus*
- *Ilex* (several species)
- *Magnolia* (several species)
- *Malus* (several species)
- *Prunus* (several species)
- *Syringa* (several species)
- *Viburnum* (several species)
- *Zelkova serrata; Z. sinica*

Tipshoot Cuttings

If you're looking for the absolute easiest means of asexually propagating plants, this is it. To take cuttings, you'll need a sharp knife (a pruning knife is best, although a single-edged razor blade will also work); a container with a clear glass or plastic-bag cover (or a propagating case, discussed later in this chapter); some coarse sand mixed evenly with peat moss, and a root-inducing powder.

Softwood or Summertime Cuttings

From mid-May until sometime in July, most trees and shrubs send out new growth. By cutting off some of this new growth — called "tipshoots" — at the proper time in late spring or early summer, you can increase the number of trees and shrubs around your home with very little effort. The key phrase here is "proper time."

Expert propagators use a simple test to tell when a softwood shoot is ready for propagation. If a shoot bends but doesn't snap, it's too young; if it bends and snaps partway through, it's too old. If it bends and snaps cleanly (like a ripe spear of asparagus), the time is perfect. In general, the best cuttings are those in which the sap has begun to flow, which usually means in early spring, although some plants do just as well from cuttings taken in fall. Some experimentation and a little luck will help you determine the best time for taking your cuttings.

When your shoot is ready for propagation, sever it with the pruning knife, making a good, clean cut just below a node. The cutting should be around 5 inches long. Quickly remove the lower leaves on the cutting and place the sprig in a pot of cool water to keep it from drying out. Even a couple of minutes of exposure to air may damage the cutting and prevent it from rooting.

After collecting all the cuttings you want, dab their bases with a paper towel and dip them into the root-inducing hormone powder according to directions on the package. Then moisten the rooting medium, punch holes into the soil with a sharpened pencil tip, and insert the sprigs. With the eraser or your fingers, gently but firmly tamp the soil around the base of the cuttings to remove all air pockets. Sprinkle lightly (a fine mist is best), cover with a clear plastic bag or glass pane, and place in indirect light. Do not place in direct sunlight or your cuttings will cook!

Keep the medium moist but not saturated. Ventilate by perforating the plastic bag in several places or by tipping up the glass cover for an hour or so each day to discourage the formation of mold.

Once the cutting is placed in the soil, the cells around the cut will grow in an effort to heal the wound, resulting in the formation of a callus. When the cut surface is covered, roots will "strike" or begin to form. In time, the roots will grow thick enough to support the plant. That's when the new plant can be moved to a small container of its own.

How long is "in time"? Depending upon the plant, the roots should strike from 2 weeks to several months. Some of the easiest plants to propagate with tipshoots are ficus, fuchsia, and hibiscus.

Hardwood or Wintertime Cuttings

Many plants, including evergreens such as *Taxus, Juniperus, Chamaecyparis,* and *Thuja,* can be rooted from cuttings made during October, November, and December, when the plant is dormant. Such cuttings are called "hardwood cuttings." It's particularly effective for the narrow- or flat-leaved coniferous species such as *Arborvitae, Juniperus* (juniper), and *Cupressus* (cypress). The procedure is identical to that for softwood cuttings.

Once the roots have formed, proceed with caution. It's easier to lose a young plantlet at this state than at any other time during the propagation process. The most serious damage is done when well-intentioned but inexperienced gardeners take their fragile new plantlets to a sunny windowsill for the "best" possible light. Unfortunately, a new cutting receiving too much sun will lose too much water through transpiration, shrivel up, and die. Instead, move your young plantlets to brighter locations only gradually as they continue to grow and harden off. Mist them often until they're several weeks old and able to endure a regular watering routine. Remember that these young plants are fragile. Treat them gently until they're tough enough to survive on their own.

Cutting Methods

Various ways of taking cuttings from a plant and turning them into new plants make propagating an extremely rewarding pastime. Where else can you buy a single item and end up with 5 or 10 or 50 more for virtually no additional investment? That's exactly where taking cuttings comes into play. Here are a few of the different methods available to you.

Leaf Petiole

Remove a leaf with up to 1½ inches of the petiole (the stalk that attaches the leaf to the stem). Insert the lower end of the petiole into the growing medium. One or more new plants will form at the base of the petiole. The new plants are then severed from the original leaf-petiole cutting, and the cutting may be used again to produce more plants. Plants that can be propagated by leaf-petiole cuttings include African violet, *Peperomia, Episcia, Hoya,* and *Sedum.*

No Leaf Petiole

This method is used for plants with thick fleshy leaves. The snake plant (*Sansevieria*), a monocot or plant that grows by deposits on its inside, can be propagated by cutting the long leaves into 3- to 4-inch sections. Insert the cuttings vertically into the medium. The African violet, a dicot or plant that grows by deposits on its outside, can be also propagated from the leaf blade. Cut a leaf from a plant and remove the petiole. Insert the base of the leaf vertically into the medium, making sure that the main vein (the mid-vein) is buried in the rooting medium from which new plants will spring.

Split Vein

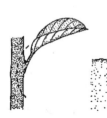

Detach a leaf from a rex begonia and remove the petiole. Make cuts on several prominent veins on the underside of the leaf. Lay the leaf, bottom side down, on the medium. If the leaf curls up, hold it flat by covering the margins with rooting medium. New plants will form at each cut. A variation of this method is to cut the leaf into wedges, so that each piece has a main vein. Insert the leaf wedge into the medium with the main vein partially covered. Other plants that can be propagated using the split-vein technique include gloxinias and temple bells.

Leaf-bud Cuttings

Leaf-bud cuttings are used for many trailing vines and where space or cutting material is limited. Each node on a stem can be treated as a cutting. This type of cutting consists of a leaf blade, petiole, and a short piece of stem with an attached axillary bud. Place cuttings in the medium with the bud covered by up to 1 inch of soil, leaving the leaf exposed. Plants that can be propagated in this manner include clematis, rhododendron, camellia, jade plant, rubber plant, devil's ivy, grape ivy, *Dracaena*, blackberry, *Mahonia*, and heart-leaf philodendron.

Cane Cuttings

Cane cuttings provide an easy way to propagate some overgrown, leggy house-plants such as dumb cane, corn plant, Chinese evergreen, and others with thick stems. Cut a leafless section of stem 2 to 3 inches long from an older stem. Each cane should have one or two nodes. Lay the cutting horizontally on the medium or insert vertically with about half of the cutting below the surface of the medium. Make sure a bud is facing upward. Pot the plantlet when roots and new shoots appear.

Offset

Some plants, such as strawberry bego-nias and spider plants, send out runners with small plantlets on the ends. You can produce new plants from these "children" either by snipping off the runner and placing each plantlet in growing medium or by tucking each plantlet into the grow-ing medium and snipping off the runner after the children take root. Either way, you won't have to wait long before you've turned one large plant into several new ones.

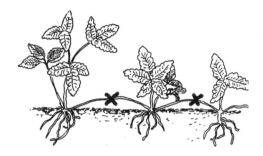

Soil Layering

Another way to propagate plants with flexible stems is to bend the stem down toward the soil in which the plant is growing. Secure it with a wire hoop and cover the stem and hoop with soil. Eventually, the stem will strike roots and send up a new plantlet. When it's sturdy enough, sever the stem from the parent plant and repot the child in its own container. Plants that take well to layering include climbing or hanging plants such as *stephanotis* and passion flower.

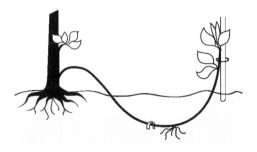

Using a Propagating Case

If you're serious about plant propagation, you should consider buying or building a propagating case — a large waterproof box with a removable clear plastic or glass top.

You can make a temporary propagating case by lining a large cardboard box with a plastic bag (any color will do). Cut a second piece of clear plastic large enough to cover the top of the box and attach it with tape or snap-type clothespins. Fill the box with several inches of sand, vermiculite, or a mixture of the two, dampen, and you're all set. Once the cuttings are inserted in the box, keep the case sealed to prevent the plants from drying out. Roll back the plastic wrap partially for an hour or so a day to permit air circulation and prevent mold, and keep away from direct sunlight.

If you'd like to build a permanent, more durable case, you'll need some lumber and a suitable place to work. You can build the case to any dimensions, although it should be small enough to be manageable, perhaps 3 feet wide by 2 feet deep and 1 foot high.

A permanent propagating case consists of a clear-plastic top supported by a wooden frame. Use 1-by-2s to make the frame as well as the framework for the lid. Line the inside of the box with waterproof plastic such as heavy-duty trash bags, drop cloths, or even pond liner. Then cover the lid framework with clear plastic. Set the lid on top of the box, and place the entire frame in a brightly lit area, away from direct sunlight.

Fill the case with several inches of dampened rooting medium (sand, vermiculite, or a combination of the two), and plant your cuttings. Prop the top open for an hour or so each day to prevent the young cuttings from rotting. After 1 to 3 months, you should see several sturdy new plants ready for transplanting into their own containers.

If you're not a do-it-yourself, you can buy a clear-plastic storage bin with a top that can be propped open for an hour or so each day and prepare it as above.

Not Just for Cuttings

Besides starting your cuttings in the propagating case, you might also choose to start your seeds in it. Since it retains moisture well, it provides an excellent greenhouse-like atmosphere for tiny seedlings to sprout. Just remember to give them plenty of bright light (without burning them with direct sunlight!), and keep the rooting medium constantly moist but not saturated. Feel the soil often, and, when it seems to be drying out, sprinkle it lightly or mist until it's moist again. Remember: Cuttings won't root and seeds won't germinate in a dry growing medium, but neither will they live for long after sprouting if the medium is saturated. Those tender young roots require well-oxygenated soil in which to grow.

When your new cuttings and seedlings are ready for transplanting, remove them from the propagating case, and replant them into pots about 4 inches in diameter. As the plants continue to grow, transplant them into their permanent containers.

Science Says

The most popular means of propagating plants, according to the North Carolina State Extension, is via cuttings. For greatest success, they should be taken from the current or past season's growth, depending upon the plant. After taking the cuttings, remove any flowers and flower buds so that each cutting's energy can go toward producing new roots instead of developing flowers. Take the cuttings only from disease-free plants, preferably from the upper part, the newest growth.

On its website, the Extension advises, "The fertility status of the stock [parent] plant can influence rooting. Avoid taking cuttings from plants that show symptoms of mineral nutrient deficiency. Conversely, plants that have been fertilized heavily, particularly with nitrogen, may not root well. The stock plant should not be under moisture stress. In general, cuttings taken from young plants root in higher percentages than cuttings taken from older, more mature plants. Cuttings from lateral shoots often root better than cuttings from terminal shoots."

When is the best time of day to take cuttings? "Early morning is the best," according to the Extension, "because the plant is fully [fluid]. It is important to keep the cuttings cool and moist until they are stuck. An ice chest or dark plastic bag with wet paper towels may be used to store cuttings. If there will be a delay in sticking cuttings, store them in a plastic bag in a refrigerator."[2]

While the Extension goes on to say that the terminal parts or tips of the stem produce the best cuttings, a long shoot can be divided into several cuttings from 4 to 6 inches long. To create a cutting from a shoot, use a sharp thin-bladed pocket knife, pruning shears, or single-edged razor blade. Dip the cutting tool in rubbing alcohol or a mixture of 1 part bleach to 9 parts water to prevent transmitting diseases between parts of the plant.

On plants with small leaves, remove the leaves from the lower one-third of the cutting. On large-leaved plants, remove leaves from the lower third, and cut half of the remaining leaves away in order

to reduce water loss through the plant's process of transpiration. The extension adds:

> Treating cuttings with root-promoting compounds can be a valuable tool in stimulating rooting of some plants that might otherwise be difficult to root. Prevent possible contamination of the entire supply of rooting hormone by putting some in a separate container before treating cuttings. Any material that remains after treatment should be discarded and not returned to the original container. Be sure to tap the cuttings to remove excess hormone when using a powder formulation.
>
> The rooting medium should be sterile, low in fertility, and well-drained to provide sufficient aeration. It should also retain enough moisture so that watering does not have to be done too frequently. Materials commonly used are *coarse* sand, a mixture of 1 part peat and 1 part perlite (by volume), or 1 part peat and 1 part coarse sand (by volume). Vermiculite by itself is not recommended because it compacts and tends to hold too much moisture. Media should be watered while being used.[3]

To put a cutting into the growing medium, make a hole with a sharp pencil and insert from one-third to one-half its length into the medium. Tamp the medium down around the cutting to remove any large air pockets. Space cuttings just far enough apart to allow all leaves to receive sunlight. Then cover the cuttings with plastic and place in indirect light. Keep the medium moist until the cuttings have rooted.

The time required for your cuttings to root, according to the Extension, "varies with the type of cutting, the species being rooted, and environmental conditions. [See chart, "Optimum stage of tissue (wood) maturity for rooting stem cuttings of selected woody ornamentals."[4]] Conifers require more time than broadleaf plants. Late fall or early winter is a good time to root conifers. Once rooted, they may be left in the rooting structure until spring."[5]

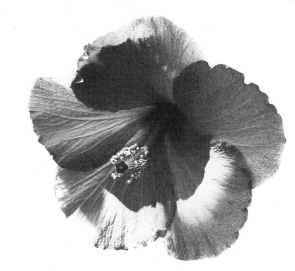

Chapter Twelve:

Special Needs for Fruiting Plants

THERE ARE NO HARD AND FAST RULES for growing trees and shrubs with special needs — and by that, I mean primarily fruiting plants. But to be successful at getting your indoor plants to bloom and set fruit, you'll need to provide them with the proper growing conditions.

As with any plants, some fruiting plants are easier to grow than others. I've found plants such as bananas (*Musa*) and pineapples (*Ananas*) easy to grow and to induce to bear inside under a fairly wide range of conditions. Both of these are warm-climate plants that adapt well to year-round indoor growth. Some people have told me they've successfully brought various species of blueberry (*Vaccinium*) to fruit indoors in an acidic soil of around 5.0 pH, but I've never tried that. One of the more trying fruiting trees I've known is the common apple (*Malus*). It's a hardy enough tree that blooms profusely outdoors from its third year on, and certainly there are enough species and varieties — including dwarfs — to satisfy the indoor grower. But turning blooms into fruit is another story.

To begin with, apple trees, along with blueberries and some other flowering plants, are for the most part self-sterile. That means the pollen of one tree will not fertilize the pistils of the same tree. To produce fruit, cross-fertilization of two or more trees is necessary. Thus, to induce apple trees and other self-sterile trees to bear fruit indoors, you must grow at least two trees (and preferably more) in the same room.

Secondly, since apple trees (and all flowering trees and shrubs) normally require wind or insects such as bees to complete pollination, the indoor gardener without these two agents must take over the job himself. With self-fertile plants, the pollen can be spread from flower to pistil by shaking the plant periodically while it is in bloom. With such self-sterile trees as apples, though, you must take a small brush and gently dust the blooms of one tree and then those of another, thus transferring the pollen between the two plants. This procedure requires more than a little time and patience each day that the plants are in bloom — and apples may have blooms for 2 or 3 weeks each spring.

The last and most peculiarly trying aspect of bringing apple trees in particular to bear indoors, concerns temperature. In subtropical climates (and that includes your living room which is something of an artificial subtropical climate normally ranging from 68°F in the winter to 90°F or more in non-air-conditioned homes in the summer), apple trees bloom but don't set fruit. Studies have shown that winter temperatures must average below 48°F for 4 months if the apple tree is to complete its rest period, which is crucial to producing fruit. Unless you're an Inuit, that could create some serious problems for you with your family.

There are ways to beat the game, if you're game enough yourself. If you have an unheated garage and live where winters are cold enough, you can move your apple trees there for wintering. Just make sure the thermometer in the garage doesn't plunge too low, or the roots may suffer freeze burn in their relatively shallow

containers. Also, be sure to water the plants lightly perhaps once a month, even though the trees are dormant. And if the temperature plummets to 32°F or lower, wrap their containers in burlap or straw to help insulate against hard freezes.

As the temperature begins to warm in March, gradually acclimate the trees to their summer surroundings and increase the amount and frequency of watering in keeping with their growth.

Beyond apples, all fruiting plants require more nutrients during their flowering period than at any other time of year. But they require the right nutrients in the right proportions. Plants fed a food too high in nitrogen will divert their efforts from producing flowers (and, later, fruit) to producing additional foliage. In order to prevent that, adjust the diet of your flowering trees and shrubs several weeks before flowering is expected. Reduce their intake of nitrogen-rich food and increase their intake of phosphorus-rich food, which is necessary for a healthy production of flower buds.

There are, as we have discussed, numerous fertilizers comprising a wide range of minerals and elements available commercially. Throughout the growing season, I generally feed my foliage plants a mixture of decomposing organic matter: carrot shavings, potato peels, ground apple cores, chopped orange skins, coffee grounds, and whatever other vegetable matter I can find. Occasionally, once every 2 months or so, I subsidize this food with a full dose of Miracle-Gro™ 15-30-15, according to directions for houseplants. From 1 to 2 months before my flowering trees and shrubs are due to bloom, I curtail the use of mulch and rely exclusively on the commercial food supplemented by a little bone meal (0-12-0). But, even though the directions on the package call for ½ teaspoon of Miracle-Gro™ to 2 quarts of water applied every 3 or 4 weeks, I give my plants half the dosage — ¼ teaspoon to 2 quarts of water applied twice as often, that is, every 10 days to 2 weeks. The Miracle-Gro™ has twice as much phosphorus (30 percent) as nitrogen (15 percent), so the fertilizer encourages my plants to produce flowers at the expense of excessive foliar growth.

After the plants have finished flowering or fruiting, I return to my original feeding program of mulch and occasional applications of Miracle-Gro™. Why Miracle-Gro™ when so many other products are on the market? For the best reason I know of — it works. I'm not saying something else wouldn't work just as effectively for you, and I'm not discouraging you from finding it. But, since I'm personally satisfied with the results of my feeding program, I'll stick to it. However, sometime in the future I may try feeding my flowering plants a commercial food containing *three* times as much phosphorus as nitrogen, a 10-30-10 formula, for example. Experimentation, after all, is one of the joys of life, no less so with growing plants than with anything else.

Light and Water

Many people find their flowering trees and shrubs produce plenty of flower buds that fall to the ground before they ever have a chance to open. Or the buds may open perfectly and then shrivel up and fall off before pollination occurs. In these cases, the cause is probably one of two culprits: insufficient light or too much water.

When a plant enters its flowering stage, it needs plenty of full-spectrum light, that is, light containing all the rays in the natural spectrum of the sun, including ultraviolet. Make sure your flowering plants receive from 14 to 16 hours of sunlight a day during their flowering seasons, or supplement the natural light with some of the many grow lights available commercially.

That other bogeyman, too much water, can be equally damaging to flowering plants. But flowering plants actually require more deeper waterings than their foliar brethren. I know I've been preaching to go easy on the watering of your potted plants, and that's a sermon I'm going to stick with. But during flowering season, watering once a plant's soil begins to dry out requires a good soaking. Water as if there's no tomorrow, and then allow the soil to dry out again before repeating in a week or so.

Just how moist a "good soaking" is requires an answer only you can give. It's not as tough a task as it sounds once you've gained a little experience. Generally, when the soil is dry to the touch or the plant makes its thirst known by turning down its leaves slightly, it's time to water until the excess flows out of the drainage hole. Remove any sitting water, and you'll be good as gold. Just remember that both flowers and fruit drain the plant of water far more quickly than foliar growth does; so, keep a watchful eye on the soil and the plant.

Pruning

Apple, orange, lemon, lime, tangerine, and fig trees all need to be shaped by pruning from their first years as saplings. It's during those early years, the years prior to fruiting, that the trees take on their general form, which they'll maintain for the rest of their life.

When a fruit tree reaches maturity, however, it will need special care in pruning in order to produce the most fruit possible from one season to the next. Here's a short guide.

Apple. A popular container plant, dwarf apple trees produce most of the fruit at the tips of the spurs formed on two-year-old branches, so you must be careful not to remove these spurs in pruning. Many spurs that have been dormant for a year or more will suddenly begin fruiting. If you cut away even those spurs that don't seem to be productive, you may actually decrease the amount of fruit your apple trees yield. New growth should be pruned, but after the tree has reached satisfactory proportions to encourage heavier fruiting on the spurs of the older wood.

Orange. Head back only as necessary to keep growth in proper proportion. No additional pruning is necessary once bearing stage is reached.

Lemon. Without constant check, lemon trees grow long and scraggly. Keep them headed back to a neat, full form.

Tangerine. Head back as with orange.

Lime. Head back as with orange.

Fig. One type of fig, *Calimyrna*, doesn't readily produce lateral branches near the trunk, choosing instead to send out an open framework that may, in time, look awkward. Head back the scaffold branches to force lateral branch growth and a fuller, bushier look growing closer to the trunk.

For more detailed information on pruning, see Chapter 14.

The Best Fruiting Plants

If you have a spacious, airy sunroom, conservatory, foyer, or great room, some of the best fruiting plants you can grow include figs, citrus fruits, apricots, peaches, and grapes.

Peach and Nectarine. Natural or genetically dwarf varieties are best. Check out bonanza (peach) and nectarella (nectarine) that can bear fruit on 30-inch stems. Keep them in a well-lit, sunny spot and provide plenty of ventilation in warm weather.

Apricot. Popular compact varieties include Shipleys and Goldcot, both highly productive container plants in direct sun. Supply good drainage and hand pollinate with a Q-Tip or soft artist's brush to ensure setting of fruit.

Mulberry. This slow-growing tree makes a great specimen in a large room with bright indirect light.

Ground Cherry. Try *Prunus angulate* for its petite tomato-like flowers and cherry-sized red fruits in attractive paper-like husks. Prolific bearer when grown in pots larger than 1 foot in diameter.

Pomegranate. Try the compact *Punica granatum* Nana, growing to 3 feet high. Although the plant produces attractive fruits in fall, they rarely ripen indoors. Grown more for visual effect.

Fig. A good fruiting plant that thinks it's a vine even while you treat it as a tree. *Negro largo* does well with roots confined in a large pot, although you may need to prune it heavily to keep it from getting too rambunctious.

Calamondin Orange. This tree, *Citrofutnella mitis variegate*, is a cross between a kumquat and an orange. Its variegated foliage and small sour fruit make for a colorful year-round display.

Pineapple. The *Ananas comosus* makes a good, easy-to-grow plant from a nursery specimen or from scratch simply by planting the top of a commercial fruit. The plant can reach up to 6 feet high and spread nearly as wide.

Lemon. The dwarf Meyer lemon, or *Citrus x meyeri*, requires a slightly acidic soil and full sun, preferably southern exposure. Lemon trees require 12 hours of light during winter, so you may need to supplement with a grow light.

Science Says

According to the University of Florida IFAS Extension, you should encounter few problems in growing fruiting trees and shrubs in containers provided you pay attention to these major requirements of the plants:

- **Water.** Most container-grown fruiting plants fail for one reason: overwatering. Plants growing in containers should be watered only as needed. For most plants, the upper surface of the soil should be allowed to become dry to the touch before watering. Then water thoroughly by slowly filling the container. Good drainage of excess water from the containers is essential. Cool growing conditions generally slows plant growth and thus reduce the plant's need for moisture, so watering should be less frequent.

- **Light.** Most fruit crops grow best in full sunlight, although some tolerate partial shade. Remember that plants grow in direct proportion to the amount of light received, all other variables being equal, so container-grown fruiting trees and shrubs should be placed where they will receive maximum sunlight. And don't subject your plants to drastic changes in light exposures, i.e., plants growing in partial shade should not be suddenly exposed to full sunlight. Moving plants from outdoors to indoors and vice-versa should be done gradually.

- **Fertilizer.** Good nutrition is essential for the success of container-grown fruit trees, but excess fertilizer can result in overgrowth, poor fruiting, and possible dieback due to salt accumulation. Water-soluble fertilizers are widely available and should be used according to label directions. If mature foliage is a deep green in most plants, adequate fertilizer is being used. Many fertilizers can be used successfully provided they are complete and balanced. They should contain nitrogen, phosphorus, and potassium in balanced proportions and lesser amounts or traces of magnesium, iron, manganese, zinc, and copper. The ingredients and quantities of each nutrient contained are listed on the fertilizer label. Salt accumulation indicated by a white crust on the soil or container may be due to excess fertilization or water containing considerable soluble salts. Such containers should be thoroughly leached by slowly running water through the container for several minutes. This will wash excess salts down through the soil and out the drainage holes.

- **Pruning.** With few exceptions, fruit trees will develop and maintain their natural shape with little or no training or pruning. If a plant does become "leggy," those branches should be cut back partially to force new interior branching and bushiness. If the top growth exceeds the capability of the root system, some leaf shed and twig dieback may occur. Such plants should be headed back heavily to rejuvenate them. When plants are heavily pruned, less fertilizer and water will be necessary to compensate for the reduced plant size.

The Extension concludes with some general notes on fruiting:

> Most fruit crops will produce fruit in containers, given time, good care, and adequate size and age. However, naturally large fruit trees will require larger containers to bear much fruit, as the amount of fruit produced is proportional to the plant's size, so large yields should not be expected. Many fruit plants need to be quite large in order to fruit at all, so their size can quickly become limiting [factors] in containers.[1]

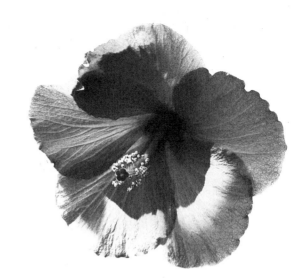

Chapter Thirteen:

Companion Planting for Health

Nᴏᴛ ᴛʜᴀᴛ ʟᴏɴɢ ᴀɢᴏ, a person's home medicine cabinet consisted not of a mirror-faced box filled with iodine, hydrogen peroxide, and castor oil, but of potted plants. Millennia before the American Medical Association existed, Socrates was prescribing cures for people's aches and pains by using commonly available botanicals. Today, those same medicinal plants are still growing freely, and if you teach your family how to rely upon them, you won't ever have to worry about running out of some commercially available medicinals again. Aloe vera, for example, is used throughout the world for everything from salving minor burns and bruises to cleansing and purifying the skin. I can't count the number of times I burned myself in the kitchen and turned to an aloe leaf to deaden the pain. And that's just the beginning.

Horticulturist, Heal Thyself

Today's most popular medicinal treatments have existed practically forever. From marijuana to catnip, there are hundreds of remarkably common herbs, flowers, berries, seeds, and plants that serve all kinds of medicinal and health purposes that might surprise you: anti-inflammatory, antifungal, insect repellent, antiseptic, expectorant, antibacterial, detoxifying agent, fever reducer, antihistamine, pain reliever, and much more. They can be grown alone in pots or in combinations with the trees and shrubs you already have growing in your home (or will have shortly!). All provide differing health benefits. Here are several potent plants you can find in the wild, in your own backyard, or in your local nursery. Note: Before utilizing any medicinal plants, be sure to check with a physician or licensed holistic practitioner. Medicinal plants are just what the name implies — medicine. As such, they may cause adverse reactions in some people and might interact or interfere with prescription medicines.

- **Marijuana.** Aside from the tittering reaction this word often generates, the pot plant has been used for medicinal purposes for centuries. In fact, hemp from the marijuana plant was George Washington's primary and Thomas Jefferson's secondary crop. The Declaration of Independence was written on hemp "paper," as was the Gutenberg Bible. Before being banned as a "hard drug" until that stigma was lifted in 1970, medicinal marijuana was used worldwide as a wonder drug. Today, its legality throughout North America is steadily expanding. Besides offering a limitless, renewable resource in the form of foodstuffs and products challenging cotton and plastic, its health benefits include relief from depression, reduced anxiety, reduction of blood pressure, pain management, and the treatment of glaucoma. Numerous dwarf varieties are available and ideal for companion planting.[1] Before seeking to grow or even possess marijuana — either plants or seeds — make certain you know what the pot laws are in your state or local jurisdiction.

- **Ferns.** Among the world's oldest plants, lady and bracken ferns, can ease the pain from stinging nettle and poison ivy, and reduce discomfort from minor cuts, stings, and burns. Simply grab a few fronds and roll them up between your palms to produce a juicy pulp to rub onto the wound. Since most ferns prefer high humidity, avoid attempting to grow in dry environments.
- **Mint.** Most varieties of mint, including spearmint, Korean mint, apple mint, and peppermint, are used to help soothe headaches, fight nausea, calm the stomach, and reduce nervousness and fatigue. Korean mint, also called Indian mint and hyssop, is also used as an antiviral, making it useful for fighting colds and flu.
- **Catnip.** The "bad boy" of the animal kingdom is renowned for driving cats wild. This member of the mint family can relieve cold symptoms and break a fever while inducing sweating. Catnip also helps stop excessive bleeding and swelling when applied topically. It's reportedly useful in treating gas, stomach aches, and migraines. Catnip can also stimulate uterine contractions and thus should be avoided by pregnant women.
- **Alfalfa.** Long known as a widely heralded fodder for livestock, this ground cover is inexorably rich in minerals and healthful nutrients and other elements.

Its roots grow from 20 to 30 feet deep, making it a hardy plant during periods of drought. It's also remarkably high in protein for a plant. Originally found in the Mediterranean and Middle East, its use is now worldwide — and no longer confined to animal husbandry. People have used it for decades to cure morning sickness, nausea, kidney stones, kidney pain, and urinary-tract infections. It's a strong diuretic with slight stimulant power, which can come in handy on the heels of a prolonged illness. It's also a liver and bowel cleanser and can even help reduce cholesterol when used over a long period. Easy to grow from seeds or transplants and use as a tea.

- **Sage.** Another incredibly useful herb, sage is anti-inflammatory, antioxidant, anti-carcinogenic, and antifungal. Its scientific name, *Salvia officinalis*, is derived from the Latin word *salvere*, which means "to be saved." It was once used as a preservative for meat before refrigeration. Among other things, sage aids in digestion, relieves cramps, reduces diarrhea, dries up phlegm, fights colds, reduces inflammation and swelling, and acts as a salve for cuts and burns while killing bacteria. It is also alleged to restore color back to gray hair.
- **Blackberry.** Everyone knows and appreciates the tasty little fruits from this hardy multi-caning plant, loaded with antioxidants and vitamins, but fewer people realize how healthy the roots and leaves are, as well. Native Americans used the stems and leaves for healing, while savoring the tender young shoots as a vegetable. The dried leaves and roots make a tea useful in the treatment for dysentery and diarrhea, as well as serving as an anti-inflammatory and astringent. It's ideal for treating cuts and inflammation in the mouth. A dwarf variety named "Baby Cakes" is thornless and ideal for container growing as a companion plant.[2]
- **Wild Quinine.** Herbalists throughout the United States and Europe have been using this prolific herb for years to treat diseases such as lymphatic congestion, colds, ear infections, sore throat, fever, general infection, and Epstein-Barr virus. The tops of the plant have a medicinal "quinine-like" bitterness used to treat intermittent fevers, which has earned the plant its name.[3]
- **Sweet Marjoram.** Although slightly different than oregano, the two are often used interchangeably. The Greeks called it the "Joy of the Mountain" and revered the plant throughout the Mediterranean for its fragrance, flavor, and medicinal qualities. The herb has many uses, including as a digestive aid, but it's also a top-notch antifungal, antibacterial, and disinfectant.

- **Burdock.** The use of burdock as both a food and a medicine extend back hundreds of years. Europeans used the plant as an herbal medicine. The Chinese and East Indians used it for lessening the severity of colds and flu. Native Americans used it to treat rheumatism, while Shaker communities used it to treat gout, syphilis, and leprosy.[4] On her website, garden writer Karen Bergeron relayed: "An old time herbalist, now deceased, told me that the seeds of Cocklebur [burdock] soaked in milk will cure cancer."[5]

- **Sweet Violet.** Native to Europe and Asia, sweet violet is grown worldwide for its delicate form and flowers. More than a pretty face, it is brewed down into a thick syrup to treat colds, flu, coughs, and sore throat. As a tea, it's used for relieving headaches and muscle and body pain.

- **Plantain.** Not to be mistaken for the tropical fruit commonly used in cooking, this plant is often regarded as a weed today, but it's actually one of the most revered healing herbs in the world. The plant takes its name from the French, meaning "sole of the foot," after the shape of the plant's leaves. To this day, those greens are used to treat bites, stings, cuts, sore feet, and ailments of the eyes, tongue, and mouth. Plantain is also a nutritious wild edible that is high in calcium and vitamins A, C, and K.[6]

The young tender leaves can be eaten raw in a salad, while the older stringier leaves can be boiled in soups and stews. A must-have for any medicinal gardener.

Other Popular Companions

All these healthful companion plants bring up the question: For which trees and shrubs do these plants make good company? That answer, you'll be pleased to know, is as wide as the great outdoors brought inside. Known for centuries as plants that assist in the growth of other plants, these and other companion plants do so in the wild by attracting beneficial insects, repelling pests, and providing nutrients, shade, and support. Today's indoor gardener more often looks for companion plants to fill the gaps beneath a tree or shrub and the edge of the pot while looking attractive in the process.

While not all companion plants will grow equally well with all trees and shrubs, most do. And for those that don't, you can always transplant your medicinal herbs and other companion plants into their own smaller pots to intersperse among your larger potted trees and shrubs — or even grow outdoors where you'll still get all the benefits of centuries of natural medicinal remedies.

Of course, not all companion plants need be medicinals. Many ornamentals make excellent companion plants, as well, including spreading alyssum, begonias, holy basil, petunias, and strawberry plants. All add a splash of color and texture to a planting while coexisting quite comfortably with most larger potted plants.

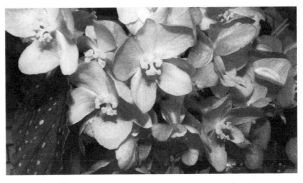

Begonia.
PIXABAY

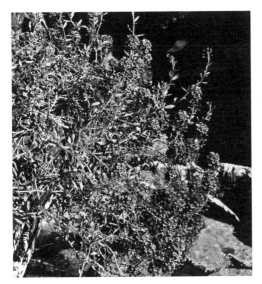

Alyssum. HERDA

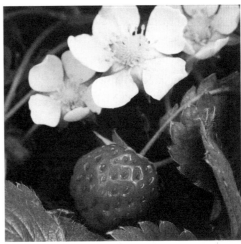

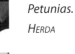

Petunias.
HERDA

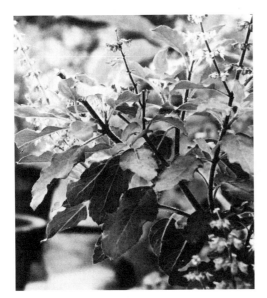

Holy basil. USDA

Strawberry.
PIXABAY

And don't overlook the possibility of growing various foodstuffs as companion plants for your trees and shrubs. Particularly attractive are above-ground plants such as compact bush peppers, bush tomatoes, okra, lettuce, kale, chicory, and dwarf anythings. Avoid the root vegetables such as potatoes and carrots though, for their underground growth will interfere with the roots of their larger roommates.

Science Says

Although the term *companion planting* extends most frequently to the field of agriculture where different plants are interspersed to promote higher fruit and vegetable yields (planting nitrogen-inducing beans alongside nitrogen-depleting corn, for example, makes good sense), it can also apply to indoor gardening. Even though the purposes for companion planting outdoors versus indoors are different, the results can be similar in that combining two or more different plants in the same container produces a more aesthetic "finished" look to the indoor garden. Indoor companion plants also generate an electrical field that, while not detectable to humans, is widely detected by insects and, especially, other plants and may offer a burgeoning new industry in the near future.

According to a Stanford University study released in 2010, "Stanford engineers discovered a means of generating electrical current by tapping into the electron activity in individual algae cells.

Photosynthesis excites electrons, which can then be turned into an electrical current using a specially designed gold electrode. This study could be the first step toward carbon-free electricity directly from plants."[7]

These electrical impulses may also help spur plants in close proximity to one another to respond by growing larger, faster, and healthier than their solitary neighbors.

While the list of companion plants and those host plants that aid one another in growth and production is long and, undoubtedly, debatable, one person's negative experience may well be another's success. The nice thing about using companion plants in your container garden is that, if something doesn't work for you, you can dig it up and replace it with something that does.

For a relatively exhaustive list of companion plant vegetables, fruits, herbs, and flowers used in the field, check out this Wiki[8] entry.

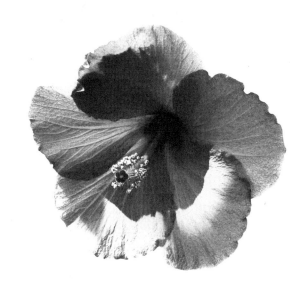

Chapter Fourteen:

Pruning and Heading Back

"PRUNING" IS A STRANGE WORD with even stranger connotations. It comes from the medieval French *proignier*, meaning "to cut off superfluous twigs, branches, and shoots." To most beginning gardeners, it means trouble.

I imagine only a handful of gardeners out of every hundred or so understands the necessity of pruning trees and shrubs to keep them healthy and under control. Fewer still know the basic rules and tools for successful pruning, not to mention the terminology associated with the ancient art.

At the mere mention of the word, many gardeners panic, conjuring up images of Mr. Brown — a middle-aged man balding at the crown and dressed in baggy pants, baseball jacket, and tennis shoes — running electric shears over a row of outdoor hedges. In 20 minutes flat, he has carved away two-thirds of the shrubs'

growth, dumped the twigs in the trash, and hung the shears in the garage for use again next fall before plopping down in front of the television to await the coming of winter.

That's not pruning. It's murder.

Others envision Mr. Jones who lives right down the block from Mr. Brown. He spends the entire spring cutting his outdoor shrubs and trees into perfect geometrical shapes — domes, triangles, squares, hearts, cats, dogs — so that, by summer, his lawn looks like a box of Lucky Charms.

Still others, like Mr. Smith, view pruning as a lot of hooey. After all, Mother Nature put the plants here on Earth. Certainly she can take better care of them than we can.

Well, Mr. Smith is wrong on two counts. In the first place, whatever shrubs and trees Mother Nature deposited on

Mr. Smith's property were in all likelihood thinned or removed by man in his never-ending quest for expansion. Thick forests were reduced to thin groves and then to occasional specimens and finally to barren fields as bulldozers and shovels clawed their way across the countryside. In the end, municipal employees and private citizens reintroduced most of their preferred trees and shrubs after home construction had ground to a halt. Mother Nature had nothing to do with that vegetation. At best, she was an adoptive parent.

Secondly, plants left to their own devices certainly can do quite well for themselves. Lightning, wind, animals, insects, and diseases "prune" broken or spindly limbs or even entire plants. In that way, the weak perish and the strong grow stronger.

Unfortunately, man doesn't usually live in harmony with the woods and forests. His desires within his own community don't often correspond with the will of Mother Nature. Mr. Smith doesn't want a backyard that looks like an untouched National Forest. He wants shade trees tall enough to walk under without bending.

He may also want grass, a flower garden, vegetables growing off to one side, a few fruit tree espaliers lined neatly against the garage, a bird bath, a patio, and perhaps a small herb garden right outside the kitchen door. Mother Nature can't work miracles.

Likewise, the pruning approaches of Mr. Brown and Mr. Jones leave something to be desired. Their attack is wasteful and aesthetically defeating. There's nothing either useful or attractive about uniformly clipped shrubs or plants indiscriminately shaped regardless of their natural form.

Fortunately, there is a better way. And what you learn and put into practice on your indoor trees and shrubs will be invaluable to you as you work with your own landscape, both indoors and out.

To the indoor gardener, pruning is as important and necessary a procedure as watering, feeding, and repotting. Once certain principles and procedures are learned, it's certainly no more difficult than confronting a store full of plant foods and fertilizers and trying to determine which is best for you. But first, you must understand the very basic objectives of pruning.

Objectives

The most efficient pruning practice is one that modifies the growth of a plant to meet your immediate objectives without destroying the natural growth pattern or appearance of the plant. With very little effort, you can turn a beautiful and leafy *Ficus benjamina* into a scraggily, misshapen twig. All it takes is a pair of pruning shears and the proper amount of ignorance.

Some indoor plants require less pruning than others in order to meet your immediate or long-range goals. Some, in fact, require none. (Don't get too excited; there aren't many of those around!) Other plants, depending on their natural growth habit, require almost constant effort. You'll want to avoid the plants in that group unless you have plenty of time and patience (and just a touch of masochism) to devote to them.

Maintaining Plant Health. The first and most important objective in pruning indoor trees and shrubs is eliminating all diseased, broken, or dead wood. Easy enough. The reason you want the bad wood gone is that, if left alone long enough, it could host and spread disease to healthy growth or allow disease to enter through wounds that could eventually destroy the plant. Pruning is an effective preventive.

Eliminating Undesirable Growth. Trees and shrubs force-grown within the strict confines of a pot often tend to put out unattractive, awkward, or even unhealthy growth. Pruning away all crossing branches, for instance, prevents possible rubbing and injury to the plant, while at the same time opening up the inside of the plant's structure to allow more light to penetrate. This is a very desirable benefit to the plant, especially indoors, where it may have to struggle to receive enough light. Thinning out weak, scraggly, or worn-out branches is also important and can likewise improve the overall health of the plant, the quality of future foliage, and — in the case of flowering plants — the number and vitality of their blooms. Pruning, too, is invaluable for maintaining the desired shape of the plant, which should be in keeping with its natural growth tendency.

Removing Sprouts and Suckers. By removing any shoots that come up next to the main plant, you'll accomplish two things at once: strengthen the main plant by eliminating competition for water and nutrients and create a new plant for repotting, if desired. In order to remove an offshoot, you may have to brush back some of the soil or even dig a little to expose the runner that connects it to the main plant before snipping it off.

Controlling Plant Growth. Perhaps the most obvious objective in pruning indoor shrubs and trees is to prevent them from growing through the roof, which can make things messy when it rains. Pruning does prevent plants from putting out too much undesirable growth, but, in addition, such surgery actually stimulates additional growth where it belongs — which is wherever you want it. In this sense, pruning is a bit like cavorting with the gods: you feel an intense sense of power and pride in being able to alter, speed up, or slow down the growth of your plants in whatever direction you desire. However, the rewards do not come without some effort.

Since indoor plants are totally removed from their natural environment, they're dependent upon you for life. The same home or even the same room may shelter a selection of trees and shrubs from such divergent places as Madagascar, Burma, Australia, Greece, China, our own Rocky Mountains, and the southern and midwestern United States. These specimens are so removed from their natural habitats (which may include plateaus, mountains, forests, or deserts) that it's no wonder their growth may be sluggish, weak, or even nonexistent at first. Careful, knowledgeable pruning habits can help restore some of the natural growth and vigor these plants enjoy in their natural environment.

Topping Trees

One word of caution when it comes to topping trees (cutting back the main leading branch): Don't! At least not with deciduous or coniferous trees. That's the prevailing conventional wisdom. By cutting back the leader (the highest point that usually grows from the plant's main trunk), you can shock the plant to the point where it may never recover. While plants naturally heal-over lower, lateral- or side-branch cuts, they don't have that ability with leaders. Lopping off the leader of a tree can also expose the tree to insect, fungal, and bacterial attacks that may eventually prove fatal.

You can, however, top certain tropical plants (plants that cannot withstand cold temperatures) to maintain their height or spur new top growth. I regularly top plants such as ponytail palms and yuccas. In fact, most tropical plants that grow on a single stalk can be made to increase their top shoots by cutting them back by as much as a fourth. (You can insert the pruned cutting into a rooting hormone and plant it to attempt to get it to grow, although success rates vary depending upon a number of conditions, as discussed in Chapter 11.) Within a few weeks, depending upon the plant and growing conditions, you may see several new plantlets sprouting from the section of the headed-back trunk just below the cut. Those plantlets will eventually grow into a fuller, more luxuriant, healthy-looking tree.

Pruning's Effects on Plants

To understand pruning's effects on a tree or shrub, you need to understand what takes place inside the plant. A typical tree or shrub is composed of four elements: root system, trunk and branch framework, leaves, and propagating or seed-producing flowers. All these elements combine rather amazingly to produce growth. Yet each plays a unique role in the development of the plant.

Roots

These thin, fibrous, underground extensions serve as an anchor for the plant, holding it upright and in place. But they do much more than that.

The growth of a plant is an integrated phenomenon that depends on a proper balance and functioning of all parts. If a large portion of the root system is destroyed, a corresponding portion of the leaves and branches will die. If a tree's aerial growth is continually cut back, some of its roots will die. Proper functioning of roots is as essential to the processes of photosynthesis as are the leaves and other chlorophyll-bearing parts of the plant. Typical roots are the sites of production of essential nitrogenous compounds that are transported up through the woody tissues of the plant, along with water and mineral nutrients.

The fine feeder roots of a plant are connected to the leaves by an elaborate

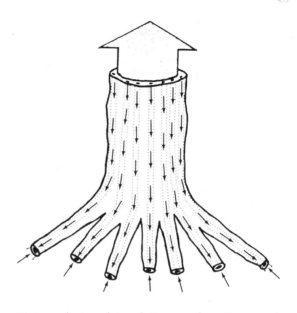

Water and minerals in solution pass from the ground into the roots and throughout the trunk, branches, and leaves via the core. Food manufactured through photosynthesis returns from the leaves to the roots via a layer under the bark known as the cambium.

plumbing system consisting of larger transport roots, trunk, branches, and twigs. Like the plumbing in your home, if part of the system gets blocked off or destroyed, the entire system may be affected.

Trunk and Branch Framework

All plants except microscopic ones have a main stem structure. This consists, in most varieties, of a central trunk with auxiliary branches and sub-branches and is similar in appearance to a well-developed root system. Like roots, branches

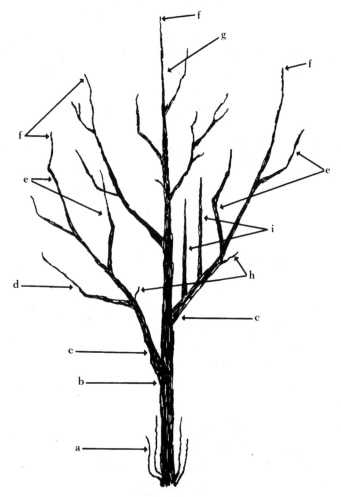

The pruning terminology for a plant's framework — its growth above ground: a) suckers; b) narrow or weak crotch inclined to split as tree matures; c) primary scaffold branches; d) secondary scaffold branch; e) lateral branches that grow from primary and secondary scaffold branches; f) terminal growth that includes all growth from the end of a branch; g) leader that is taller than all other branches; h) spurs or short lateral branches that bear the fruit on many fruiting trees; i) waterspouts.

serve a double function. They hold the plant erect and in balance, and they act as a plumbing system, like our own veins and arteries, constantly moving matter up and down between different parts of the body. In plants, water and minerals percolate upward through the core, or center, of the trunk and branches, and manufactured food seeps down through a membrane-like layer just beneath the bark, called the *cambium.*

Since, in our discussion of pruning, we'll be referring to certain terms, you should learn their meanings. The *leader* is the name given to the one dominant branch that points skyward, usually a continuation of the trunk. *Scaffold branches* are the main side branches, usually the best-developed branches on the plant. *Lateral branches,* which grow off the scaffolds, are shorter, smaller branches. *Spurs* are the very short branches, more like stubs, that carry leaves, flowers, or fruit.

Leaves

These fantastic "food factories" use energy from the sun to help absorb carbon dioxide from the air and combine it with water percolated up from the roots to form sugars and starches that sustain the plant's growth. Other substances from the roots combine with chlorophyll in the leaves to play a role in this reaction. Each leaf consists of a *broad blade,* which is connected to a branch by means of a *petiole* or stalk.

Under normal conditions, a plant has just enough roots to provide the leaves with raw materials to manufacture food. But when roots are reduced in volume, as when a tree is dug up for transplanting indoors, those remaining are incapable of sending up the same amount of food-producing solution. As a result, the amount of foliage above ground is reduced by dying off. The dead foliage requires still less work of the roots, which in turn send up even less solution. Thus, whenever a plant's root system is reduced, the framework and leaves of the plant are affected, sometimes permanently.

To prevent dieback when transplanting trees and shrubs that have sustained some root damage, you need to prune back the foliage proportionately in order to maintain healthy, growing, well-balanced plants. This is one of the core concepts of pruning and one of the most important things to remember: When a plant's roots are reduced in volume, the plant's foliage must be reduced proportionately. Otherwise, the plant will be out of balance, suffer, and possibly die.

Flowers

The flowers of most plants are attached to the branches. Their only goal is to create seeds for the species to perpetuate itself. Without the flowers, most trees and shrubs would soon perish. Once properly pollinated, the blossoms produce seed, varying from a microscopic speck to an avocado or a mango seed or the giant seed of the coconut palm.

Not all trees' flowers, remember, are conspicuous or decorative. Some are so small or inconspicuous to be nearly impossible to discern from a distance of even a foot or two.

Growth Cycle

Each of these four plant parts functions efficiently on cue. At different times of year, roots, stems, leaves, and flowers go to work in different ways to accomplish different goals.

Springtime is the start of most plants' growing season. Food that had been stored away in the roots and branches suddenly begins to flow. Roots begin a new season of growth, too, as buds swell and burst open, and branches, leaves, and flowers come to life.

If the plant is deciduous — sheds its leaves in fall — it puts out all new foliar growth in the spring. If evergreen —a cone-bearing tree or a flower-bearing plant such as rhododendron or other tropical evergreen — it adds new growth to existing foliage.

Initially, spring growth is slow. The first few leaves come from buds formed the previous year. These new leaves immediately begin producing food to supplement the plant's stored food, which the new growth is gradually depleting. Finally, the plant sprouts enough leaves to sustain itself, and the source of food for growth shifts, almost as if a breaker had been thrown, from previously stored to currently manufactured.

The plant continues to grow throughout summer and generally into fall. At the onset of cooler weather and other signals, even indoor plants sense the shifting of the seasons to cooler, shorter days and gradually stop putting out growth. The roots remain active, though, absorbing life-sustaining nutrients and water to see the plant through the approaching winter months of dormancy and into the new spring and summer months of growth.

In their dormant stage, water, food, and any supplemental light you normally give your plants should be reduced, and they should be kept at a cooler temperature when possible. Plants will remain lethargic — much like hibernating bears — until the arrival of spring signals once again the beginning of their growth cycle.

Bud Growth

A bud is the point on the stalk where, given sufficient stimulation and proper growing conditions, a new branch will begin to develop. It's important to be able

to recognize a bud, because they tell many things about the plant, including what you can expect if you prune the plant at any given location.

The terminology for buds is relatively simple. *Terminal buds* grow from the ends, or terminals, of branches. *Lateral buds* grow behind terminal buds on a branch. *Dormant buds* are simply buds that are not yet ready to respond to growth stimuli. They are generally smaller and less developed than terminal or lateral buds.

Where to Cut

There's only one proper place to cut back, or "head," the terminal branches of shrubs or trees to reduce their girth and slow their growth: that's immediately above a good, healthy, well-developed bud. Here's what you can expect to happen when you make such a cut in a branch.

In general, cutting back a branch affects only the growth of those buds in the immediate vicinity of the cut. If you make two cuts on the tree, the following three things will happen.

- From the top bud (the new terminal bud) on each stub, a new stem develops even though the dormant buds on each stem below the point of pruning remain inactive.
- Each new branch grows enough to maintain the balance of the tree. The

branch on the left, from which you cut 6 inches, grows back 6 inches plus another foot or so to keep up with the growth of the tree as a whole. The branch on the right, from which you cut 3 feet, grows back 3 feet plus another foot or so to keep up with the growth of the tree. Therefore, the cut on the left branch stimulates a foot-and-a-half of new growth. The cut on the right branch stimulates 4 feet of new growth.

- The 4 feet of new growth on the right produce many strong buds and new leaves. The foot-and-a-half of new growth on the left produces smaller buds and fewer leaves. That's because more of the plant's food and growth hormones are directed to the side of the tree that has suffered the most damage (received the heaviest pruning) at the expense of the left side of the tree, which receives only minimal amounts of food and growth hormones. Other factors, too, come into play. But the important thing to remember is: The more severe the pruning, the more the plant will respond to that pruning.

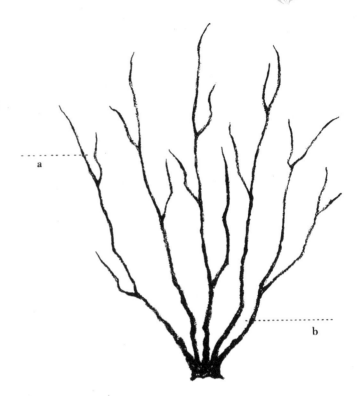

The effects of pruning can be seen in this illustration. The left-hand branch, pruned to point "a," will produce growth equivalent to that pruned away plus a modest amount more. The right-hand branch, pruned to point "b," will produce growth equivalent to that pruned away — a much greater amount than with the left-hand branch — plus a modest amount more. This is an example of how heavier pruning produces more new growth than light pruning.

Besides stimulating a plant's new growth through pruning, a smart grower can also determine the direction of the new growth. Look closely at the buds on a plant. Large or small, each one points in a particular direction. Either that direction is toward the center of the tree (an inside bud) or away from the center of the tree (an outside bud). The way that bud is pointing is the direction in which the new branch will grow.

Knowing this, you can determine not only the direction in which a new branch will grow but also the purpose of that new growth. By pruning to an inside bud, you can make a new branch grow in toward the center of the tree and thus fill in any weak spots or gaps in the tree's structure. Such pruning also reduces new outward growth or crown "spread" by directing the energy of the plant's growth inward. By pruning to an outside bud, you can make a branch grow outward and increase the general spread of the plant while avoiding crowding the inside framework.

Heading Back Versus Thinning Out

The two basic pruning techniques are known as *heading back* and *thinning out*. Heading back consists of cutting back a branch to a bud, most often to control the size, growth rate, and growth direction of a plant. Thinning out is the *complete removal* of branches by cutting them away at the main trunk or a lateral branch. Such thinned branches rarely grow back.

By comparison, heading back to a nearby bud usually results in a fuller, bushier plant because the cuts, as we saw, stimulate new growth from the new

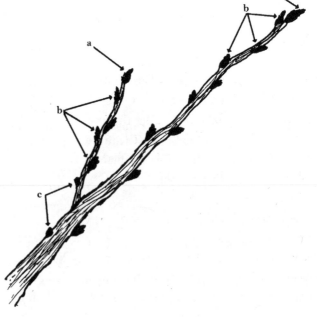

Bud terminology and bud growth direction: a) terminal buds, b) lateral buds, c) dormant or undeveloped buds. As one bud is pruned away, the new terminal bud will produce growth in the direction of the bud's tip.

terminal bud. Thinning out produces the opposite effect. Such pruning opens up spaces within the framework of the plant and makes the plant airier. Whether you thin out or head back depends strictly on the results you want to achieve in your pruning and how you want the plant to respond.

Summer Versus Winter Pruning

Light heading back (minor pruning) can be done at any time of year without harm to a plant, but heavier pruning should come at definite points in its annual growth cycle.

Deciduous plants should generally be pruned in winter when they are dormant. At that time, leaf-holding stems and branches are inactive because the foliage has dropped, and the trees are feeding lightly from food stored in the roots. That's the best time to prune back whatever wood you find undesirable.

Conversely, deciduous plants should not be pruned severely during the summer months because that's the time when the plants are working to produce food not only for growth but also for storage for the coming winter. They need those leaves during summer! If you greatly reduce the foliage at that time, the plants will be unable to produce and store enough food to see them through winter and next spring's growth push. As a result, their growth will be reduced or completely stunted.

Light summer pruning is valuable for maples and other trees that bleed profusely if pruned in late winter or early spring when the sap is flowing strongest. Pruning such trees in the fall or early winter, after food has been stored and before sap begins to flow, is best.

Conifers, too, are best pruned lightly in summer while the new growth is soft and short, although light pruning in winter will not harm the trees.

Summer pruning is best, too, for flowering shrubs and trees where winter pruning would remove much of the bloom-supporting wood, resulting in fewer blossoms the following season. So, wait until the blooming period is over (sometime in early summer) before pruning your flowering plants.

Whether you follow a practice of light summer pruning or somewhat heavier winter pruning, remember not to clip too much from the plant at any one time. The prudent pruner adheres to the mandate of architect Ludwig Mies van der Rohe: Less is more.

It's not how much you remove from a tree or shrub, but what you remove, when you remove it, and where you remove it from that counts.

Science Says

Pruning trees and shrubs is both an art and a science. From an aesthetic perspective, a practiced eye is needed to evaluate a plant and determine what pruning it needs to achieve the desired appearance. From a scientific perspective, knowing the when, where, and how of pruning is equally important.

Of course, following a "Right Plant, Right Place'" approach to choosing plants for the home or office helps many gardeners avoid unnecessary and repetitive pruning tasks. On its website, the Clemson University College of Agriculture, Forestry and Life Sciences says:

> Why create a problem when it could be avoided altogether? In using a "Right Plant, Right Place" approach, the indoor gardener should consider the site in which the plant will be placed, and then choose the plant best suited for that space. Considerations for the mature size of the plant helps to prevent plants from overgrowing their space, getting too close to structures, covering windows, obstructing doorways, etc.[1]

In the end, the decision rests with the gardener. A finely sculpted shrub or topiary is more work than most indoor gardeners have the time or patience to achieve, while allowing plants to maintain their natural form except for occasional structural and emergency pruning results in both a natural-looking and a low-maintenance homescape.

According to the College website:

> When considering the science of pruning, it's important to contemplate how pruning affects the plant. In essence, the activity of pruning causes damage and stress to the plant. In many instances, pruning is necessary to improve the health and productivity of a plant in the long term. However, a gardener should take all steps necessary to minimize the damage and stress to the plant when possible. A stressed plant is more susceptible to insect and disease attack, as well as drought and cold damage.[2]

The website goes on to categorize the three Ts of pruning: tools, timing, and technique.

Tools. Naturally, using the right tools for the job helps achieve success. Sturdy tools made from quality materials operate smoothly and efficiently. We discuss tools in more detail in the next chapter.

Timing. We covered when to prune earlier in this and other chapters. Otherwise, prune dead, diseased, and damaged wood at any time of year.

Negligence in removing these problems could expose the plant to further attack by disease or insects. Remove crossing branches that might rub against one another, causing damage.

Technique. This is the "how" of pruning, and examples vary nearly as greatly as the individuals doing the pruning.

Whenever you set about pruning, make certain you don't remove more than one-third to one-fourth of the plant's material at one sitting. Doing so can stress the plant beyond its ability to recover or to fight off insect or disease attacks.

Differences Between Shrubs and Trees

There are some inherent differences between shrubs and trees that will affect your pruning regimen. According to the University of California Cooperative Extension:

> Shrubs generally have low branches
> that arise from multiple locations near
> the soil. Trees usually have a trunk that
> branches emanate from. Shrubs usually

end up in the same form with only slight variation. Some may tend more toward a ground cover or creeping vine, but they are largely globular in form. Sometimes shrubs can be trained to resemble small trees and vice versa.

Trees have definite form that is a continuum between the *excurrent* (upright pine-tree shape) form to the *deliquescent* or *decurrent* form. The form that a plant attains is regulated by plant hormones. Although the form can be changed with pruning, the more that we try to change the innate form of a plant, the greater the pruning inputs that will be required. An understanding of the basic form of the plant will guide a natural pruning process.[3]

For these reasons, if you're not all that crazy about the prospect of learning how to prune properly, do yourself a favor and grow fewer trees and more shrubs, which are easier to maintain with a basic "haircut" than are trees.

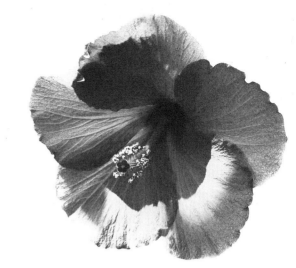

Chapter Fifteen:

Tools of the Trade

EVERY GARDENER HAS TOOLS to meet his own specific gardening requirements. But, while a complete selection varies from person to person, there are some basic tools no indoor gardener should be without.

Pruning Tools

Several firms specialize in manufacturing pruning tools. Other firms produce pruning tools as a sideline of general hardware. Both seek to protect their tools from duplication through the adoption of various patents. To the buyer, this means that each tool, no matter how similar it looks to a competitor's tool, is slightly different if only in construction or materials not readily discernible to the layman's eye. Only by using a tool for a while can you tell which pruning shears, pruning saw, or lopping shears you'll find most convenient and effective.

As pruning tools differ in style, so too do they differ in price. One word of caution: don't buy cheap. In pruning tools, cheap is far more expensive in the long run. Whereas good-quality tools will perform flawlessly and last a lifetime with only a reasonable amount of care, most bargain-priced tools will last only until you need them. Then, when the time comes for use, the spring mechanism invariably pops, or the handle cracks, or the blades don't mesh just right, and you end up sawing a limb apart. As a result, bargain-priced tools cost time, money, and very possibly your plant's life, not to mention the frustration that goes with relying upon inferior products.

Indoor gardening, luckily, requires fewer complicated pruning tools than does its outdoor counterpart. A minimum of four items, maybe five, will see you through your indoor pruning activities.

Pruning Shears. These come in two varieties, anvil and drop-forged. The anvil type has a single straight-edged blade opposite a flat bed (or anvil) of soft metal. The advantage of the anvil is that its frame is generally constructed of rolled steel or aluminum, so the tool is lighter than a drop-forged shears of similar size. In my opinion, the anvil is also hardier, a consideration if you're especially rough on tools.

The drop-forged type is the older and generally more favored of the two shears. It has a steel cutting edge along with a thicker hook and works with a scissors-like action. When in good condition, these shears make clean cuts perhaps ⅛ inch closer to the parent branch than is possible with anvil shears. The problem with drop-forged shears is that the two blades can become separated a fraction of an inch through use (or misuse, but more about that later) resulting in less efficient cutting.

Lopping Shears. For pruning branches larger than hand shears can safely or effectively handle, lopping shears come in handy. Generally, these tackle cuts up to 1½ inches in diameter with relative ease. Some cam-designed shears can go even higher. Standard care of loppers includes occasional oiling of the bearing and sharpening the blade on a whetstone.

Pruning Saw. For cuts on branches larger than 1½ inches (a rarity in indoor pruning, although with larger trees, it does occur), a pruning saw is necessary. This tool consists of a simple tapered, curved, toothed blade attached to a knifelike handle. The tool is lightweight and easily maneuverable, even in tight spots. It bites on the pull stroke instead of the push (like a common carpenter's saw) and does a fast, clean job. There's also a folding pruning saw with a handle that flips over the blade to protect the teeth. It's a useful tool to carry in your pocket while in the field or to keep neatly tucked away in a drawer until needed.

Pruning Knife. The last of the commonly encountered indoor pruning tools, the pruning knife is renowned for handling the lightest pruning needs quickly and efficiently. It has a small sharp pruning blade that's ideally built for the purpose. It, like the saw, has a curved, tapered blade leading to a knifelike handle. But unlike the saw, it is toothless. Such a knife is also handy for disbudding roses and other flowers for cut-flower table displays.

Wound Dressing. Small cuts require no special attention, but larger cuts may benefit from a covering of pruning wound dressing. This at least theoretically protects the wound and keeps out bacteria, fungi, and other disease-causing organisms while the wound slowly closes itself. Wound dressings come in many different brands. They're non-toxic and meant to be applied according to directions on the can. They are available at most nurseries and garden supply centers.

The negative side of using wound dressings is that several recent university agricultural department studies have shown them to be relatively ineffective at doing what the plant does spontaneously, that is, sealing over a wound to prevent infections. Whether you choose to use a wound dressing is solely up to you.

Care of Pruning Tools

Tools that don't work are worthless. Tools that work poorly, pulling and bruising branches that should be cut clean, are even worse. To keep your pruning tools in top condition, wipe all metal with an oily rag after each use to prevent rusting. Oil all moving parts and bearings every 6 months at least. When your tools appear to be getting dull, have a professional sharpener hone them back to their original cutting efficiency. Unless you know what you're doing, saving money by sharpening them yourself usually means unevenly honed, unsatisfactorily cutting edges.

Most of my own pruning tools are manufactured by Seymour Smith & Son, Inc. They're Snap-Cut brand, and I use them for one reason: they work.

Year after year after year. That's not to say other manufacturers' products aren't worth trying. I've heard many gardeners talk about the durability of Wiss pruning shears in particular. Others may be just as good, although I can't recommend them from personal experience. If someone you know can, that's the best reason in the world to buy them.

Additional Indoor Gardening Tools

If you plan to collect and oven-sterilize your own soil, you'll find a small sharp spade a blessing. I prefer one with a collapsible handle. You can pick one up at a camping supply shop, a hardware store, online, or (probably cheapest of all) an army surplus store. When not in use, the blade folds compactly against the handle for quick easy storage.

If much of the soil you collect is lumpy with clay or stones, you'd do well to get a medium-mesh screen to sift the dirt before sterilizing. That way, you can screen out all the undesirables before potting time. Make sure the mesh is wide enough so that small pebbles, which are good for drainage and soil porosity, and small chunks of twigs and other organic matter pass through while the larger objectionable materials are screened out. A common bricklayer's trowel is useful in pulling the soil back and forth across the screen.

Another must is a sturdy 2-gallon bucket, preferably metal, not plastic. If necessary, the metal bucket can be used in the oven as a sterilizing tin, something a plastic pail couldn't quite pull off. Make sure the bucket has a handle to aid in lugging around collected soil.

A small-capacity (about 2-quart) watering can comes in handy for watering small cuttings, seedlings, and hard-to-reach ground cover planted as companion plants to your trees and shrubs. Make sure the can has a long tapered spout for that little extra reach. To complement it, a 1- or 2-gallon sprinkling can is a must. I prefer plastic, because it's just that much lighter than metal and doesn't rust. Use this can to water your large potted trees and shrubs and, in between waterings, to age chlorinated city tap water.

Finally, no indoor gardener should be without a good sprayer or mister for adding humidity to plants. You can get anything from a $1.95 plastic quart bottle with an adjustable nozzle that lets you dial from stream to mist all the way up to a battery-operated, rechargeable electric houseplant sprayer.

Don't laugh. I have one. (Although, admittedly, when I first heard of it, I laughed.) It has become one of my favorite go-to gardening gadgets. My Hudson Cordless Electric Sprayer (manufactured by the H. D. Hudson Manufacturing Company of Chicago) is a self-contained, battery-operated spray unit that's fairly lightweight and portable. It comes with a plug-in recharger that draws little electricity and "juices up" the unit for five full hours of spraying — that's a lot of spraying on a single charge. At the flick of a switch, the device delivers anything from a steady stream to the finest mist I ever saw float out of a nozzle.

The bad news is the price. Unfortunately, it's a bit more expensive than $1.95, depending upon the capacity. Still, I find the gallon model most convenient and price-efficient. If you have a lot of plants that require frequent misting (and if you can stop laughing long enough to write out a check), I highly recommend it.

My backup sprayer is another Hudson product, a hand-compression model called the Hudson Duralite Sprayer. It sells for considerably less and delivers an equally fine mist (it has the same nozzle as the cordless electric model), but it is pump-operated, not electric.

As with other gardening implements, several manufacturers make reliable products in the sprayer-mister line. Not all are worth the price, though. I had one model that worked for only 4 months before a gasket broke and it failed to hold compression. After that, it leaked like a sieve. So buy wisely, preferably on someone's personal recommendation.

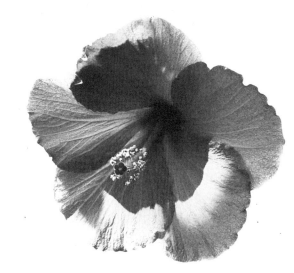

Chapter Sixteen:

Recommended Trees and Shrubs

HERE IS AN ANNOTATED LIST of trees and shrubs recommended for indoor container growth. Keep in mind the following issues while considering which plants you might want to add to your home or office.

Habit. This section tells a little about the growth pattern of the plant. It also gives general information you might find useful in considering whether or not to grow a particular plant indoors.

Flowering. If a plant is likely to flower indoors, this tells you when, what the flowers look like, and whether they are insignificant or showy.

Light and Temperature. Two of the most critical aspects of growing plants anywhere, the lighting listed here is optimal, but remember that many plants

may do nearly as well under other lighting conditions. As for the preferred temperatures, few present problems for most people who live in something other than a cave or a primitive yurt. Generally, if you're comfortable in your home, your plants will be, too. Where you may encounter trouble is if your plants are too near a door that opens and closes often during winter or a poorly sealed window that leaks cold air; cold blasts of Arctic air can cripple a tropical plant in no time. In summer, most plants don't do well when set directly in front of an air conditioning duct or unit. Similarly, if you over-summer your plants outdoors, be sure to keep an eye on both the plants' minimum temperature requirements and the overnight weather forecast as the year winds down, so you can bring them indoors before they're subject to damaging cold or frost.

Watering and Feeding. Although I describe each plant's own optimal watering preferences, don't think you have no leeway in setting up a watering schedule. If your time for plant maintenance is limited to the weekends and you'd prefer to water every Saturday morning, by all means make that your schedule. Just remember that not all plants' needs are the same. In time, you'll get to learn which need water only every other week and which can't go an entire week without water. They'll be the exception to your schedule.

The key is to check the soil condition before watering. For most plants, your index finger inserted into the soil should come out relatively dry (no soil sticking to it) to the first or second knuckle. If the finger test indicates the plant doesn't need water, skip over watering that plant that day and check back mid-week. And remember, except in those rare cases noted below, it's always better to underwater than to overwater!

Soil and Transplanting. Although some plants require a specific type of soil, most are quite satisfied with a good commercially prepared soil with a little perlite or coarse sand mixed in for additional drainage and root oxygenation. Transplanting should be done only when necessary, as when a plant shows signs of overgrowing its container. In the case of plants too large to remove and transplant into a larger pot, scrape away as much surface soil as possible without damaging the roots, and replace it with rich, fertile soil to within about 1 inch of the edge of the pot's edge, a technique called *top dressing*.

Remember that, while the advice below on transplanting is based upon the general principles concerning the plant's growth pattern, you should temper the advice with your own needs, wants, and experience. No plant has to be transplanted simply because it's getting top-heavy or outgrowing its pot. Judicious pruning of both foliar growth and roots (maintaining a balance between the two) can keep a plant virtually the same size for nearly its entire lifespan. That, in fact, is the principle behind the art of *bonsai* — growing normal-sized plants on a miniature scale. Keep in mind that, if you do repot your plant into the next larger size container filled with rich, fertile soil, it's going to continue to increase in size until it reaches its natural maximum height and width. That's a tradeoff you're going to have to make based upon your own space and requirements.

Grooming. This can be a time-consuming affair, so I suggest you conduct the majority of your pruning once a year — more often only if you have a particularly aggressive grower. Most trees require pruning in spring before the new heavy-growth season begins or in late fall/early winter after the sap has slowed down to a crawl. Most shrubs can be pruned safely all year long unless they're flowering or fruiting, in which case you'll want to wait until after the flowers or fruit have set.

Propagating. The remarks for each plant are self-explanatory.

Environment. This category takes into consideration both the plant's needs and your desires. In what environment will your plant flourish best, and what will that plant add to your home's overall décor and attractiveness?

With all that in mind, here are my picks for some of the best trees and shrubs to grow indoors.

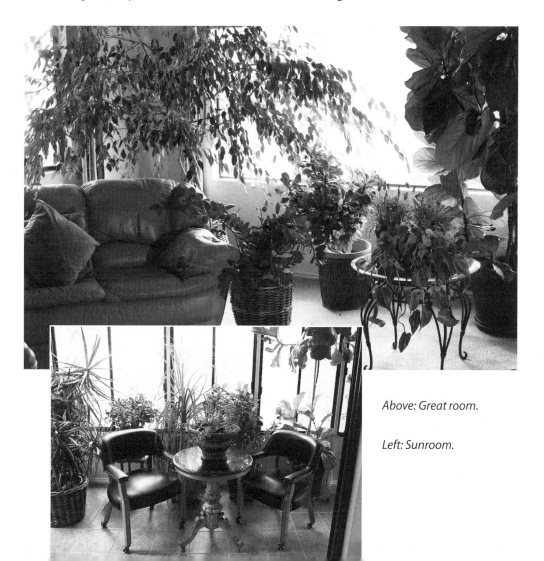

Above: Great room.

Left: Sunroom.

African Linden *Sparmannia Africana*

Habit

Fast-growing, 2 to 3 feet a year, although can be pruned and headed back to control growth. The entire plant, including the heart-shaped leaves, is covered with "hair."

Flowering

Produce a cluster of mildly scented white blooms in spring.

Light and temperature

Require a sunny spot and average room temperatures.

Watering and feeding

Check soil daily and water as appropriate; feed bimonthly during the growing season, less often during winter.

Soil and transplanting

Repot yearly as required, using a rich well-draining soil.

Grooming

May be pruned back to as much as half its size after flowering if desired to control growth.

Propagating

From cuttings taken in spring.

Environment

Given enough direct sun, its leafy green habit makes for a showy presentation in any room.

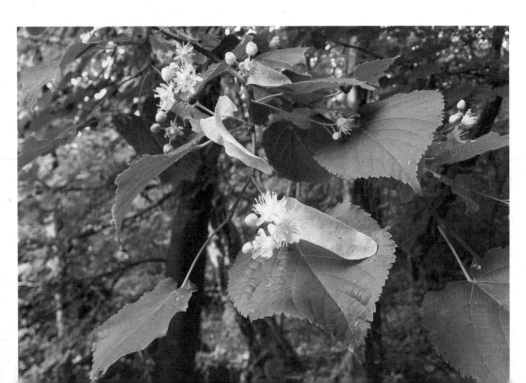

African Milk Tree *Euphorbia trigona*

Habit

Its branches reach out and up in a spreading plant that can grow as tall as 6 to 8 feet.

Flowering

Rarely receive enough light to bloom indoors.

Light and temperature

Thrive in full sun or half shade. Tolerate dry air and normal room temperatures year-round.

Watering and feeding

Water sparingly and feed lightly in summer. Water sparingly and avoid feeding during winter.

Soil and transplanting

Transplant in spring, using a well-draining planting medium. Slow growing, so repotting not necessary more than every 3 or 4 years.

Grooming

Snap off or head back unattractive shoots; otherwise, allow to grow naturally.

Propagating

Use 3- to 4-inch stem cuttings which should be dried for a week before planting.

Environment

Tolerate other plants well. Gradually work up to progressively larger pots over time.

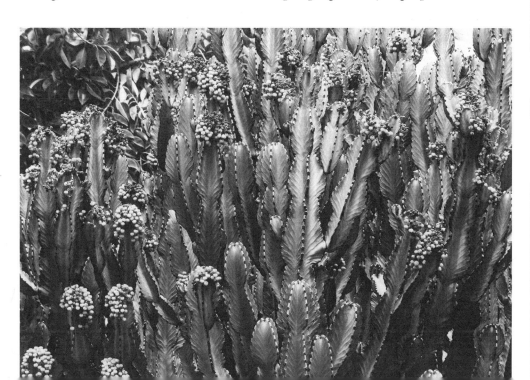

Aralia Ivy *x Fatshedera lizei*

Habit

Can be grown for years but tend to get leggy after long periods indoors. Otherwise, these actual aralia-ivy hybrids are easy to cultivate and grow. Don't branch easily on their own, tending to grow in slender columns with the leaves turned to the light. Put several plants together to appear more bush-like.

Flowering

Ivy aralia seldom flower, and since it is hybrid, it is sterile and doesn't produce seeds.

Light and temperature

Ivy aralia readily adapt to different environments, but once established, don't like to be moved. It tolerates poor lighting but can also thrive in a south-facing window where it can grow quite tall. As soon as the leaves are mature, plants can withstand temperatures down to freezing.

Watering and feeding

Undernourishment causes leaf drop from the base of the plant, so feed regularly throughout the growing period. Reduce watering in the fall to prevent excess winter growth and resume in March.

Soil and transplanting

Repot in spring as required.

Grooming

Easy to keep in shape by pruning but takes quite a while to produce new side shoots. Groom in February to encourage development of new shoots during the growing season.

Propagating

Easy to propagate by cuttings. Tip cuttings are the quickest to produce attractive new plants, but the whole stem can be cut into several two- or three-leaved sections. Plant in small pots with sphagnum moss and put pot in a plastic bag until well rooted.

Environment

Especially well-suited to positions with low or variable temperatures, e.g., as window "curtains" or on trellises.

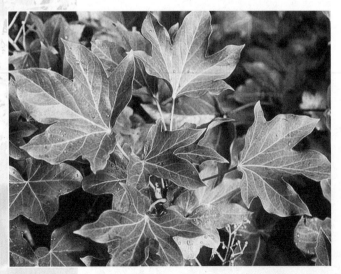

HERDA

Avocado *Persia americana*

Habit

Rarely grow taller than 4 to 5 feet indoors, putting out rapid early growth and then slowing noticeably afterward.

Flowering

The flowers have a sweet perfume-like scent but rarely develop indoors.

Light and temperature

The avocado is a high-light plant and needs as much direct southern exposure as possible. Temperatures should not fall lower than 40°F.

Watering and feeding

Keep the avocado moist, particularly during the summer growing season. Also, young growing plants should be fed regularly, according to fertilizer instructions but at least once monthly.

Soil and transplanting

Sow in light porous soil enriched with compost, shredded moss, or other organic matter.

Grooming

Leafy plants should be cut back in the spring to create a bushier plant with more side shoots.

Propagating

May easily be sown from the seeds of the fruit.

Environment

Avocado thrives best in bright, sunny exposures and gets along well with other green plants.

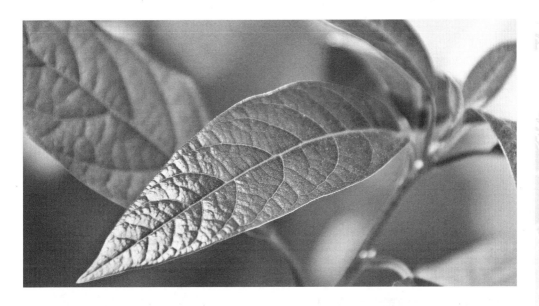

PIXABAY

Bamboo Palm *Chamaedorea seifrizii*

Habit

Grow on multiple stems from 3- to 6-feet tall indoors.

Flowering

Occasionally produce small yellow flowers along multi-branched flowering stems followed by small orange fruits.

Light and temperature

Require indirect medium to bright light but not direct sun. Normal indoor temperatures are fine for summer growth; do not expose to temperatures below 60°F.

Watering and feeding

Moderate watering and diluted liquid fertilizer during the growing season. Mist often for added humidity.

Soil and transplanting

Fast-draining, humus-rich soil works best. Repot only as required to maintain shape and size.

Grooming

Remove dying old leaves and flower stalks.

Propagating

By division in spring.

Environment

Highly prized tropical-looking foliage suitable for any decor.

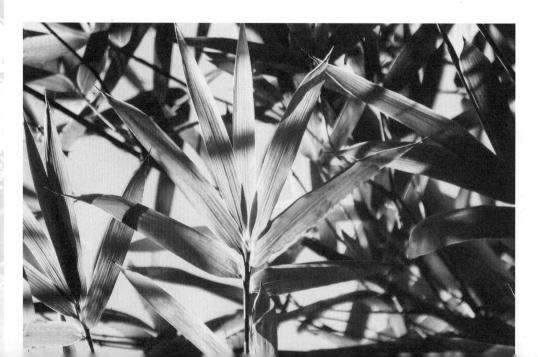

Bird of Paradise *Strelitzia reginae*

Habit

Feature lush, bluish-green leaves with a red midrib. The thick evergreen foliage resembles small banana leaves attached to long stalks but without a main trunk. Typically grow to 4 to 5 feet high and 2 to 3 feet wide.

Flowering

Emerging from the green and pink boat-shaped bracts in spring, the flowers offer petals of brilliant orange, set off by intense, blue, arrow-shaped tongues. Blooming takes place in succession over time and may continue year-round, depending upon growing conditions.

Light and temperature

Require bright direct sun but will tolerate some light shade, although flowering may be affected. Require temperatures above 50°F and preferably between 65° and 70°F.

Watering and feeding

Keep soil moist throughout growing season and cut back to allow soil to dry out between waterings in winter. Mist often for humidity. Feed bimonthly with a weak solution of liquid fertilizer throughout the growing season.

Soil and transplanting

Use a loamy, rich, well-draining soil with plenty of peat moss or leaf mold. May require an organic mulch such as leaves, pine needles, straw, or wood chips, to conserve moisture in especially dry climates. Repot as necessary when the roots show signs of overcrowding.

Grooming

Remove dead or unsightly leaves and stalks.

Propagating

By seed, suckers, or root division in spring.

Environment

Grow and thrive best as solitary container plants in direct sun and offer a majestic display of color often throughout the year.

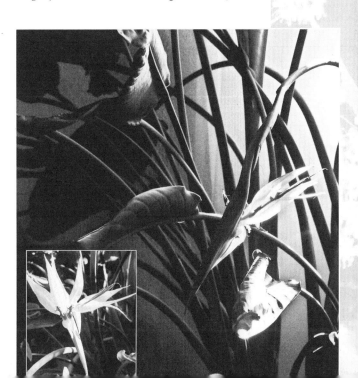

Herda

Camellia *Camellia japonica cvs.*

Habit

Camellias can grow from 4 to 7 feet tall, depending upon the variety. They make excellent shrubs.

Flowering

Flowers appear in a variety of colors and forms, although most are white or some shade of red, showy but not fragrant.

Light and temperature

Require bright indirect light away from direct sun. Plants prefer to overwinter in cool temperatures between 40° and 50°F.

Watering and feeding

Water throughout the year, including during their dormant season. Fertilize often during their growing season with a weak solution mixed with the water.

Soil and transplanting

Use a humus-rich soil with plenty of peat moss or leaf mold. Repot as necessary every 3 to 5 years.

Grooming

Rogue branches can be pruned at flowering time and put in a vase; otherwise, prune to prevent getting leggy.

Propagating

Difficult but not impossible for amateurs from cuttings or seed.

Environment

Grow and thrive best as solitary container plants.

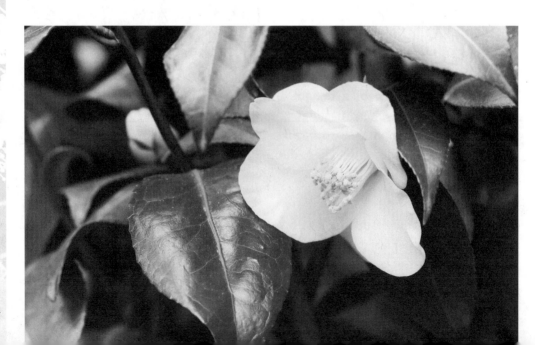

Canary Island Date Palm *Phoenix canariensis*

Habit

Delicate plants have fan-shaped leaves, reaching 6 to 7 feet at maturity.

Flowering

Inconspicuous flowers appear in groups at the base of the leaves, although rarely indoors.

Light and temperature

Protect from direct sun while young, although older plants are more tolerant. Survive high temperatures and lows down to around 46°F.

Watering and feeding

Water lightly during dormant periods and increase during active growth. Fertilize every 2 weeks during growing season.

Soil and transplanting

Repot in spring as needed. Older plants require only top dressing (surface feeding).

Grooming

Remove the first set of leaves only after the plant reaches 1 foot or more in height. Also prune out bad, dried, or withered leaves.

Propagating

Propagate from seeds that are usually exported from Spain. Occasionally, root suckers can be removed to grow new palms.

Environment

Grows well in a large tub outside in the summer. It is exceptionally hardy indoors when grown either as a specimen or a group plant.

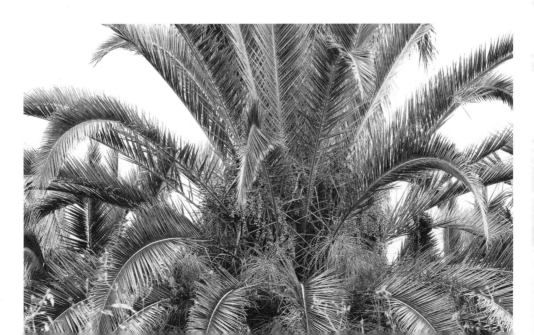

Chinese Fountain Palm (Fan Palm) *Livistona chinensis*

Habit

Grow to 15 feet or more outdoors, reaching around 4 feet indoors. Grow moderately fast at 3 to 6 inches a year.

Flowering

Rarely indoors.

Light and temperature

Appreciate bright indirect light and temperatures in the 70s throughout the growing season.

Watering and feeding

Like most palms, these require regular watering (but not soggy soil). Allow the soil to dry out somewhat between waterings. Feed container plants bimonthly with a weak liquid food in the summer only.

Soil and transplanting

Use a fast-draining potting mix and transplant only in summer when necessary.

Grooming

Remove damaged or dying fronds near the trunk.

Propagating

By seed.

Environment

Chinese fountain palms look most impressive when placed with other palms. Create a palm planting by grouping several palms together.

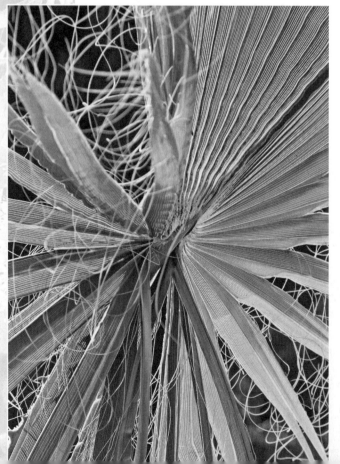

PIXABAY

Cleyera *Cleyera japonica 'Tricolor'*

Habit

A group of shrubby plants that can be made fuller by pinching back tips regularly. The variegated 'Tricolor' is commonly available and resembles the leaves of the ficus, while being somewhat more leather-like. Can reach a height of 3 feet or more.

Flowering

Produce fragrant white flowers followed by red berries in fall.

Light and temperature

Prefer bright light away from direct sunlight and can tolerate temperatures down to 45°F without experiencing adverse reactions.

Watering and feeding

Water and feed weekly during the growing season and cut back during winter. Avoid using alkaline water if possible.

Soil and transplanting

Prefer a soil comprised of equal parts peat and leaf mold with good drainage. Repot every 3 years or as required.

Grooming

Pinch back young stems to encourage bushy growth.

Propagating

Use spring cuttings and keep warm and moist until well rooted.

Environment

Fit well in most indoor settings and are easy to grow and care for.

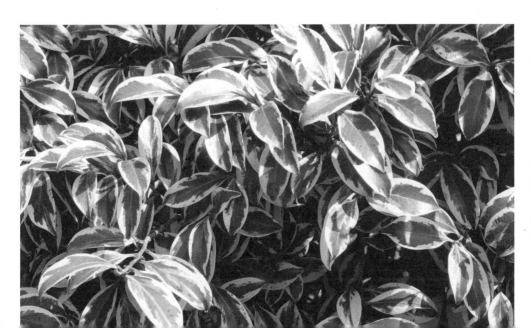

HERDA

Coconut Palm *Cocos nucifera*

Habit

Fast-growing and attractive, these produce one pair of leaves a year.

Flowering

No flowering indoors.

Light and temperature

Require strong direct sun and daily misting for humidity. Prefer 70°F temperatures or higher and winter temperatures not below 55°F.

Watering and feeding

Water thoroughly twice weekly during the growing season and once monthly during dormancy. Use liquid plant food throughout summer.

Soil and transplanting

Combine commercial potting soil with fine sand or gravel. Transplant yearly while young and switch to top dressing with fresh soil as required with mature plants.

Grooming

Trim dead or yellow tips of leaves as required, and remove bad or withered leaves at the trunk.

Propagating

Not recommended for the novice.

Environment

Definitely a singular plant, use as specimens in a sunny atrium with a high ceiling. Add ground cover to large pots if you choose.

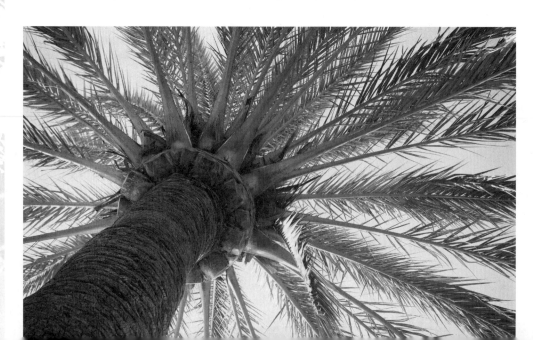

Coffee Tree *Coffea arabica*

Habit
Grow to 5 feet tall, putting on up to 1 foot of new growth a year.

Flowering
Blossom at around 3 to 4 years with white sweet-smelling flowers similar to jasmine. To encourage fruit, pollinate by hand. The berries are at first green before turning red and finally black when fully ripe.

Light and temperature
Protect from direct sun. Prefer morning or late afternoon exposures in an east- or west-facing window. Can endure winter temperatures down to 46°F but prefer normal room temperature.

Watering and feeding
Water twice weekly and mist regularly with soft water. Keep from drying out.

Fertilize with half-strength liquid plant food every other week throughout the growing season.

Soil and transplanting
Repot in spring when necessary, using a mixture of equal parts coarse sand, peat moss, and humus.

Grooming
Prune in spring as required. Save prunings for cuttings.

Propagating
The easiest way is from cuttings in spring or from seed.

Environment
Used as specimens, make excellent indoor trees.

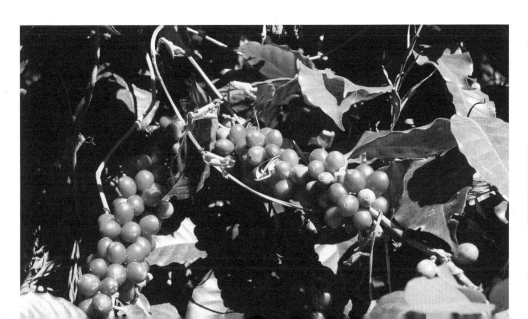

Congo Fig *Ficus lingua*

Habit
Slim, attractive plants that can reach a height of 7 feet with vertical stems and hanging wedge-shaped leaves.

Flowering
None.

Light and temperature
Prefer bright light but no direct sun and a normal indoor home temperature above 60°F.

Watering and feeding
Water well during the growing season and feed this fast grower weekly. Cut down on water during winter, but don't allow soil to dry completely.

Soil and transplanting
Do well in commercial soil with some humus added. Repot each spring as required.

Grooming
Head back for a bushier plant or to maintain proper height.

Propagating
Summer cuttings are sometimes successful.

Environment
Adds shape and drama to the indoor environment, especially when grown with weeping figs.

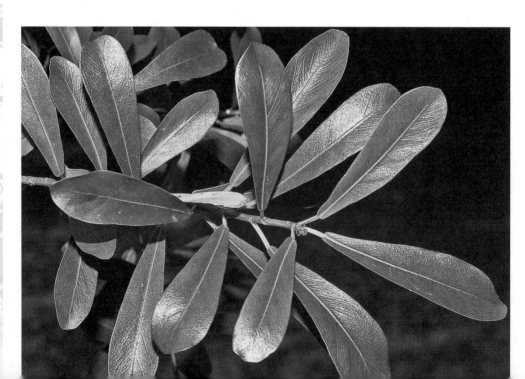

Corn Plant *Dracaena fragrans*

Habit

Normally grow to 4 to 6 feet or taller in ideal conditions. The leaves resemble those of a corn plant but with greater variegation. They are moderately slow growing indoors.

Flowering

Not indoors.

Light and temperature

Require temperatures above 60°F throughout the year and prefer bright indirect light.

Watering and feeding

Need both regular watering and feeding. Daily misting is recommended when possible but not required. Water sparingly and stop feeding in winter.

Soil and transplanting

Pot in late winter or spring using well-draining commercial soil mixed with some humus and sand.

Grooming

Control their shape by heading back and pinching side shoots as required. To revive a spindly plant, head back at a point where you'd like to see multiple tips develop and grow.

Propagating

From tip cuttings and stem cuttings. Keep cuttings warm and tented in plastic to conserve humidity until the plants have rooted and show signs of new growth.

Environment

These remarkably forgiving plants add a splash of color and visual interest wherever you grow them in areas of bright indirect light.

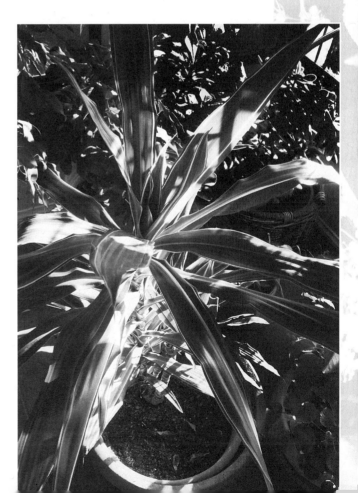

HERDA

Croton *Codiaeum variegatum*

Habit

Grow normally to 2 to 3 feet or taller in ideal conditions. Some varieties are broad-leaved, others narrow-leaved, and still others resembling the leaf of an oak. All are slow growing indoors.

Flowering

Insignificant male and female flowers grow on 4- to 8-inch stems.

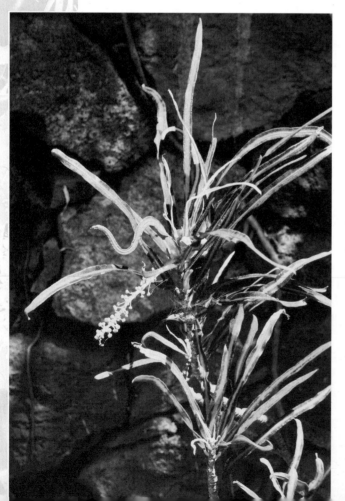

Light and temperature

Require temperatures above 60°F throughout the year and prefer bright indirect light.

Watering and feeding

Need both regular watering and feeding. Daily misting with purified room-temperature is useful. Water sparingly in winter.

Soil and transplanting

Pot in late winter or spring using commercial soil mixed with some humus and sand.

Grooming

Control the shape of the plant by heading back and pinching side shoots as required. Note: the sap may be toxic.

Propagating

From lead-shoot cuttings in spring. Keep cuttings warm and tented in plastic to conserve humidity.

Environment

Prefer high humidity, so plan on growing near other plants and misting often for a colorful, eye-catching display that adds drama to any room in the house.

Pixabay

Crown of Thorns *Euphorbia milii*

Habit

These slow-growing stemmed, exotic-looking plants are an unusual addition to any sunny place in the home. Most often mistaken for members of the cacti family, they are actually succulents.

Flowering

Prolific bloomers year-round, most often featuring reddish-orange, pink, or white quarter-inch blooms set off against glossy deep-green leaves and dark thorny stems.

Light and temperature

Love high light and even direct sun but can also live well in moderately bright settings. Survive most normal indoor temperatures but cannot live beneath 50°F, a consideration if you choose to summer the plants out of doors.

Watering and feeding

Need to dry out well between waterings. Prefer light bimonthly feedings during the growing period, slacking off on both water and food during fall/winter.

Soil and transplanting

Prefer sandy, loose, well-drained soil mixed with coarse sand or perlite. As slow growers, they need repotting only when they become too top-heavy for their existing containers.

Grooming

Remove brown or yellow leaves.

Propagating

From seed, rootings, and cuttings.

Environment

One of the simplest of plants to grow, given enough bright light, this succulent — historically associated with Christ's crown of thorns — will outperform your expectations and add a splash of color to your home. Note that the sap is moderately caustic, causing irritation with eyes or skin.

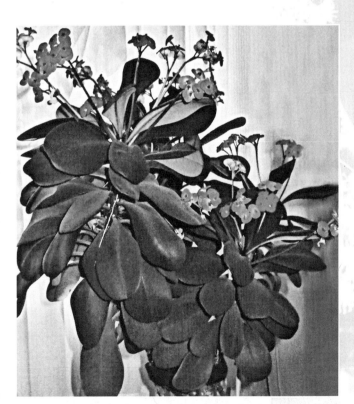

HERDA

Dieffenbachia (Dumb Cane) *Dieffenbachia amoena*

Habit

Grow to 4 to 5 feet under average conditions. The purchased plants are usually about 2 feet high, but larger specimens are sold for greenhouses.

Flowering

May flower rarely with blooms similar to those of calla lilies. The main plant usually dies after flowering but can be propagated from the numerous side shoots that spring up.

Light and temperature

Average indoor temperatures of 70° to 75° are preferable during winter, with ideal summer temperatures of around 75°F. Keep out of direct sun, since the plants grow best in partial to full shade.

Watering and feeding

Like high humidity and need to be kept damp in summer; cut back watering in winter but don't allow to dry out completely. Feed during the growing season from March to October.

Soil and transplanting

Repotting is best done in spring, using a soil blend with a high peat content.

Grooming

Prune those leaves that brown out or die off.

Propagating

Older plants lose their lower leaves, so take these stem cuttings when repotting.

Environment

Prefer high humidity and for that reason do well in the company of other plants.

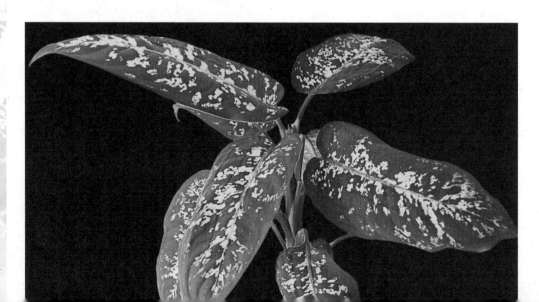

Dragon Tree *Dracaena marginata*

Habit

Reach a height of 10 feet or more if space is available. Fast growers, the best way to keep their height in check is by heading back below the existing greenery, which will produce multiple shoots to develop into new crowns.

Flowering

Virtually never indoors.

Light and temperature

Dracaenas grow best in bright light to half-shade. Can tolerate deeper shade for several months at a time before requiring more light. Overwinter at room temperature.

Watering and feeding

Water often in the summer to prevent the soil from drying out. Water sparingly in the winter. Feed once every 2 weeks during growing season.

Soil and transplanting

Do well in nearly any soil but prefer humus-rich soil mixed with a little sand. Repot when the roots begin to outgrow the container.

Grooming

Most attractive with thicker heads, which you can create by heading back the main crown below the greenery. Also look better with more than one plant in a pot.

Propagating

Rarely from seed, more often from cuttings or stem parts.

Environment

Dracaenas grow well with other plants or as solitary specimens.

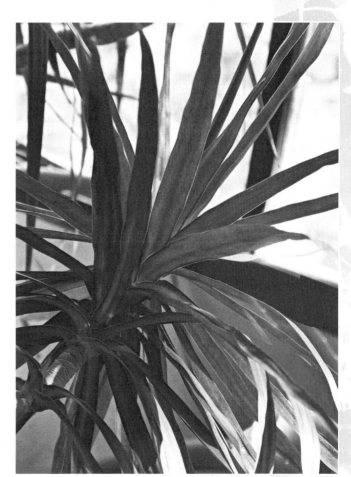

HERDA

Euonymus *Euonymus japonica*

Habit

Woody shrubs that can grow to 10 feet or taller outdoors but, by regular annual pruning, can be maintained as a full bush for indoor growth.

Flowering

Rarely indoors.

Light and temperature

Require full to partial shade and can tolerate temperatures down to 0°F.

Watering and feeding

Prefer frequent watering throughout the growing season with feeding bimonthly from spring through fall.

Soil and transplanting

Repot as required, generally every 2 to 3 years, in spring.

Grooming

Pinch back tips to encourage fuller growth. Prune in spring to maintain desired shape. Can tolerate heavy pruning.

Propagating

From cuttings made in spring.

Environment

Suitable for large containers, either indoors or outdoors as a container plant on patio or deck.

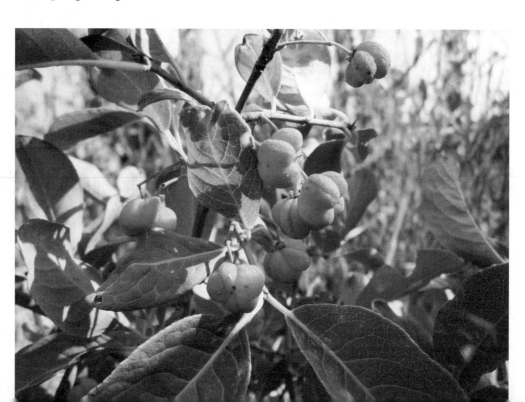

Fan Palm *Chamaerops humilis*

Habit

These low-growing wide, exotic-looking plants are definitely "space hogs" requiring plenty of room to spread out. New leaves form in summer to replace those that have died during winter.

Flowering

Insignificant, on older plants if at all.

Light and temperature

Love light but can live in more shady surroundings in cool conditions typical of the normal home setting.

Watering and feeding

Can tolerate some drought but in general should be kept moist and fed weekly through the growing season of April to October. Respond well to misting.

Soil and transplanting

Have a tendency to heave their way up out of the pot, particularly shallower containers. Repot each spring into a rich well-draining soil.

Grooming

Remove brown or yellow leaves.

Propagating

From seed or side shoots.

Environment

The easiest of all palms to grow, although space considerations must enter into play.

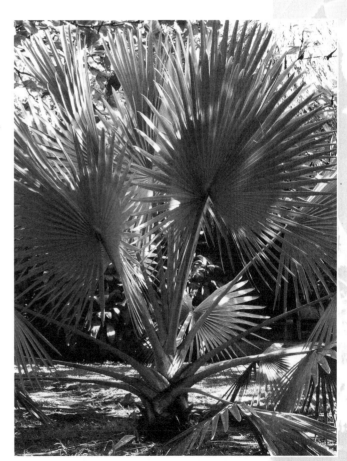

Pixabay

Fiddle-Leaf Fig *Ficus lyrata*

Habit
Evergreen plants that boast huge fiddle-shaped leaves up to 15 inches long and 10 inches wide.

Flowering
Rarely indoors.

Light and temperature
Thrive in high indirect light but never full sun. Growing to more than 50 feet in their native Amazon rainforest, they make excellent (and smaller!) container plants at normal room temperatures. Avoid exposure to cold and drafts.

Watering and feeding
Require thorough watering, but allow to dry out down to the top 1 inch of soil before watering again. Provide for good drainage. Apply liquid food at half the recommended dosage bimonthly.

Soil and transplanting
Repot one size up in early spring whenever you notice the roots growing out of the pot's drainage hole; prefer rich humus or clean peat.

Grooming
Remove dead leaves and branches and head back to maintain desired shape.

Propagating
From seeds or cuttings taken in spring.

Environment
Like most members of the *Ficus* family, these trees are actually robust vines. If allowed to grow freely, they'll take over a room. With a little attention and care, though, they make excellent and dramatic specimens.

HERDA

Fig Tree *Ficus septica*

Habit

Feature vigorous, fast growth similar to most figs with large leathery leaves and small attractive inedible fruits. Although bushy while young, older palms grow to have taller, lankier stems.

Flowering

None.

Light and temperature

Prefer indirect light to shade, making them ideal candidates for those areas too dark to accommodate many other plants. Normal room temperatures in summer work well. Plants can tolerate down to 50°F in winter.

Watering and feeding

Water bimonthly throughout the year, allowing to dry out between waterings. Use liquid plant food at half dosage with each watering during growing season and cut back in fall/winter.

Soil and transplanting

Repot every 2 to 3 years in rich fast-draining potting soil or use a top dressing as the roots begin to show above ground.

Grooming

Remove dry, brown, or spotted leaves as necessary, and head back branches to maintain desired shape.

Propagating

From seed or cuttings.

Environment

These unique and attractive trees grow well indoors and take up as much space as allowed. Their fullness makes them excellent specimen trees.

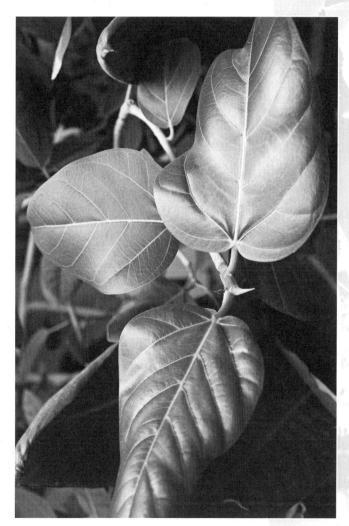

HERDA

Fishtail Palm *Caryota mitis*

Habit

Feature unique growth in the form of small triangular leaves that resemble a fish tail. Although bushy while young, older palms grow to have taller, lankier stems.

Flowering

Unlikely indoors.

Light and temperature

Prefer indirect light to shade, making them ideal plants for those areas too dark to accommodate most others. Do well in average room temperatures. Plants can tolerate down to 55°F in winter.

Watering and feeding

Water regularly throughout the year, keeping an eye on the moisture content during the growing season. Use liquid plant food at half the recommended dosage with each watering. Prefer purified water over alkaline tap water. Mist frequently with purified water to avoid brown spots from developing on the leaves.

Soil and transplanting

Repot every 2 to 3 years in rich, fast-draining potting soil.

Grooming

Remove withered leaves from base, creating a more tree-like appearance.

Propagating

From seed.

Environment

These unique and attractive palms grow well indoors in shadier spots of the home.

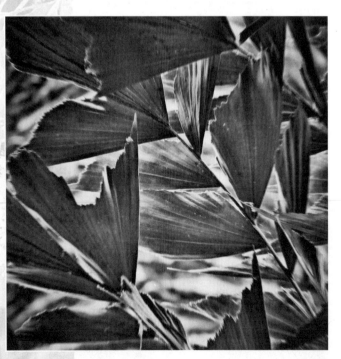

PIXABAY

Flowering Maple *Abutilon x hybridum*

Habit

Small upright shrubs with arching branches that bend under the weight of its flowers.

Flowering

Colorful flowers that look like crepe paper and bloom nearly the entire year. Flowers open up cup-shaped and flatten out in time and range from white and yellow to deep crimson.

Light and temperature

Do well above freezing, preferring temperatures above 50°F with bright direct sunlight to partial shade. Direct sun produces the most blooms.

Watering and feeding

Water when soil becomes surface-dry; do well with daily misting, but not necessary. Heavy feeders because of their prolific flower production, they prefer bimonthly feeding with half the recommended dosage.

Soil and transplanting

Repot every other spring or as required in a mixture of equal parts peat, coarse sand, and humus or leaf mold.

Grooming

Prune to maintain desired shape, usually in spring.

Propagating

By cuttings.

Environment

Because of their arching habit, make a nice choice for an entryway arbor or as potted specimen plants.

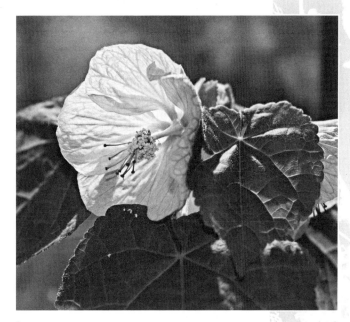

PIXABAY

Gardenia *Gardenia jasminoides*

Habit

Tight, compact, flowering evergreen shrubs with leathery leaves that grow from 2 to 3 feet high under proper conditions.

Flowering

Can flower off and on all year long but mainly in summer. The showy white flowers hare a strong perfume-like fragrance similar to that of jasmine.

Light and temperature

Prefer temperatures above 60°F. Can be forced to bloom in winter by moving to bright indirect light in August; when the flower buds appear, move to a cooler place of 60° to 65°F to delay their opening until the buds have bloomed out.

Watering and feeding

Prefer high humidity, so daily misting is a must. Maintain evenly moist soil using rain water or boiled water cooled to room temperature. Never use cold water, or you'll stunt the plants.

Soil and transplanting

Repot every other spring or as required in a mixture of equal parts peat, sand, and humus or leaf mold.

Grooming

If the plant has become leggy, it should be headed back in March or April.

Propagating

By cuttings.

Environment

Can be moved around to provide plants with optimal lighting conditions and temperatures throughout the year.

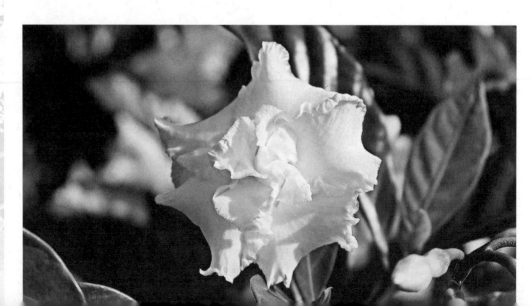

Hibiscus *Hibiscus rosa-sinensis*

Habit

Available in varying sizes, usually 6 inches to 1 foot, but they can grow to 5 feet or larger if allowed. Quick growers that require yearly pruning to keep in shape.

Flowering

Flowers range from white to deep red and appear where the leaves branch at the top of the stem, blooming for 1 to 2 days, depending on the variety. Although attractive to hummingbirds, the blooms have no particular fragrance.

Light and temperature

Like direct sun and can spend the summer indoors or out as long as the temperatures stay above 55°F.

Watering and feeding

Water regularly in the growing season, and mist during daylight hours. Feed with liquid fertilizer at half-strength during active growth.

Soil and transplanting

Use humus-rich potting soil. The best time for transplanting is in early spring.

Grooming

To stop a plant from getting too large, cut it back in early spring and remove leggy growth.

Propagation

Prepare cuttings by removing two top shoots (3 to 5 inches long) in spring. Put them in potting soil and cover with a plastic bag with air holes in it. Should develop roots in 3 to 5 weeks. Pinch back new shoots to encourage compact growth.

Environment

Maintain steady temperature and humidity as much as possible.

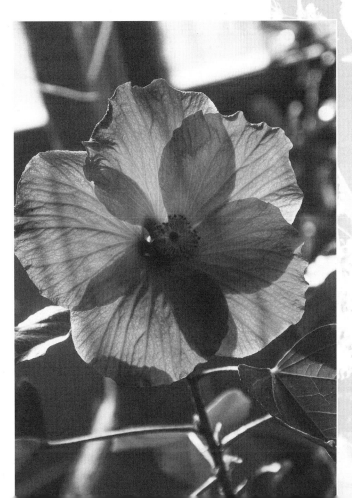

HERDA

Hydrangea *Hydrangea macrophylla*

Habit

Fast-growing shrub with broad leaves and showy flower clusters.

Flowering

Bloom from late spring through September. Flowers form on old growth (last season's wood), as opposed to new growth, so plan accordingly when pruning. Flowers range from white to blue (in acidic soil) and pink (in alkaline soil).

Light and temperature

Prefer cool, bright locations such as an east- or west-facing window. Can be set out over summer. Avoid direct sun. Overwinter best around 40°F.

Watering and feeding

Water frequently during budding and flowering (up to twice daily if outdoors during the hottest days of summer), and cut back to light periodic waterings during winter. Feed ammonium sulphate, which supplies both nitrogen and sulphur, every 2 weeks.

Soil and transplanting

They thrive best in a mixture of potting soil and sphagnum, which should be well-drained and have a pH of less than 7. Repot in January.

Grooming

Prune lightly once flowering is finished to encourage new growth that will become old growth the following year.

Propagating

Propagate with vegetative cuttings in June and July.

Environment

These showy decorative plants do well both as specimen plantings and in groups of two or more containers placed near one another.

PIXABAY

Jade Plant *Crassula argentia*

Habit

Usually small when purchased, these regal-looking plants are prolific growers when exposed to direct sun, growing to 3 feet or higher. Smaller plants begin to branch out when they reach 1 foot.

Flowering

Rarely bloom indoors unless provided with unrestricted direct southern exposure. Blooms are relatively insignificant.

Light and temperature

Have a wide range of light tolerance, although they grow best and fastest with direct exposure. Low light creates thinner stems and leaves that break off easily when touched or moved. Prevent winter exposures of 40°F and lower.

Watering and feeding

Require moisture during the growing season, but beware not to overwater. During winter, water once the leaves begin to droop or crinkle. Feed regularly during the growing season.

Soil and transplanting

Transplant when necessary in spring into a container with well-drained soil consisting of two parts potting soil and one part small gravel for drainage.

Grooming

Prune at any time if plants get too large for containers or surroundings.

Propagating

Use leaves or tip shoots partially inserted into growing medium. Very easy to propagate.

Environment

Grow well either as single specimens or several plants in a single pot.

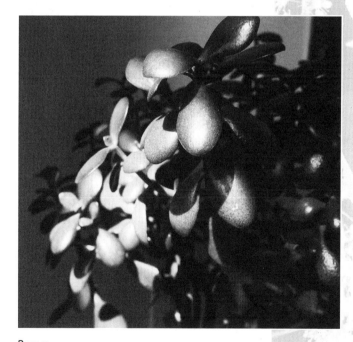

PIXABAY

Japanese Aralia *Fatsia japonica*

Habit

Large lush foliage dominates these plants that can reach 6 feet in good indirect light. These evergreens keep their attractive leaves throughout the year.

Flowering

Rarely flowers indoors.

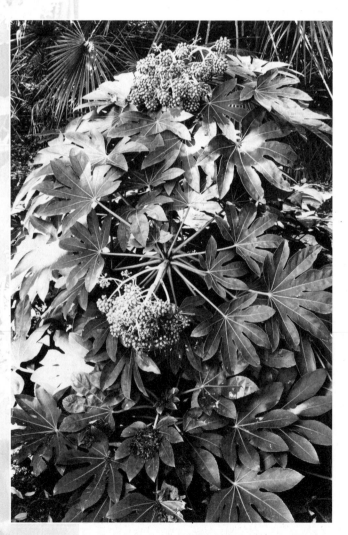

Light and temperature

Require good light, but keep away from direct exposure. Grow well in comfortable indoor temperatures. Hardy even to freezing temperatures.

Watering and feeding

Water regularly during the growing season, but avoid standing water. Feed at half the recommended rate once a month. Cut back watering during slow-growth cooler winter months.

Soil and transplanting

Thrive in rich, well-drained soils that allow the roots plenty of space for oxygen. Repot young plants annually and older larger plants only as required.

Grooming

Some heading back may rarely be required if plants get too leggy (which probably means they're not getting enough light).

Propagating

From seed or cuttings.

Environment

Beautiful specimen plants that take up plenty of space and grow well in bright indirect light. The lush glossy leaves create an ideal contrast to flowering plants, such as hydrangea, but also work well as specimen plants.

JEFF MCMILLIAN, HOSTED BY THE USDA-NRCS PLANTS DATABASE

Magnolia Tree *Magnoliaceae*

Habit

Large flowering plants featuring blossoms in white, pink, red, purple, or yellow. Magnolia trees are diverse in leaf shape and plant form and include evergreen and deciduous sorts, both tall and dwarf varieties.

Flowering

Magnificent blooms given proper growing conditions: lots of direct sun and regular feeding.

Light and Temperature

Prefer bright direct light and normal room temperatures.

Watering and Feeding

Allow the soil to dry out between watering, so oxygen can reach the roots. Prefer filtered or distilled water. Use a good water-soluble food throughout the growing season.

Soil and transplanting

Prefer commercial potting soil with added humus. Transplant only as required by the plants' growth.

Grooming

Prune away dead leaves and to maintain desired shape and height.

Propagating

By seed, air layering, or cuttings.

Environment

Between the large ovalate, glossy leaves and the magnificent large showy flowers, these plants cry out to be treated as specimens wherever enough light prevails.

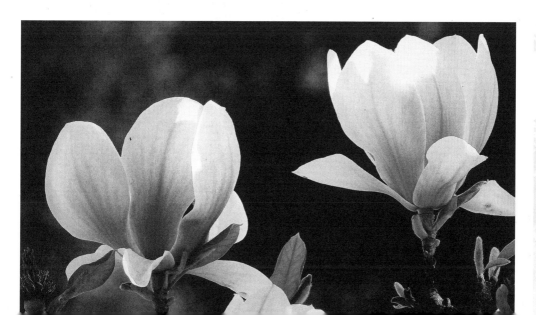

Mallet Flower *Tupidanthus calyptratus* aka *Schefflera pueckleri*

Habit

Resembling a *Schefflera*, these slow-growing robust shrubs or small trees can reach 12 feet in the wild, although container specimens rarely exceed 6 feet. Feature leathery oval, pointed leaflets on red-brown stalks in rosettes at the tip of 2-foot stalks.

Flowering

Rarely indoors.

Light and temperature

Prefer bright indirect light and normal indoor room temperatures.

Watering and feeding

Like the soil to dry out somewhat between watering, to allow for oxygen to reach the roots. Use liquid fertilizer at half the recommended dose monthly throughout the growing season.

Soil and transplanting

Do well in commercial potting soil.

Grooming

Prune as desired.

Propagating

By seed or air layering.

Environment

Tupidanthus, like its look-alike *Schefflera*, is a versatile plant that fits into a wide variety of decorator schemes anywhere throughout the home.

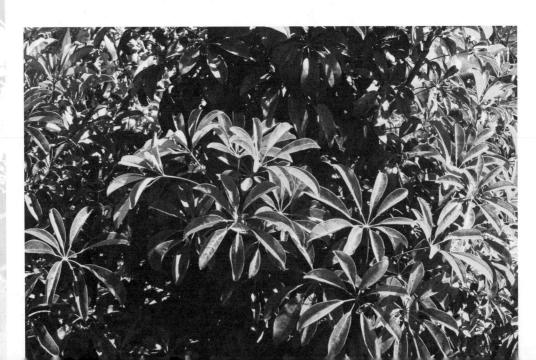

Ming Aralia *Polyscias fruiticosa 'Elegans'*

Habit

Have an upright habit, growing slowly to 4 feet or more. Look best as a multi-trunk solitary specimen. A dwarf variety growing to only 18 inches is also available.

Flowering

Rarely outside of the tropics.

Light and temperature

Prefer bright indirect light but can tolerate low light for short periods. Do well in average room temperatures above 60°F.

Watering and feeding

Keep plants moist but not saturated; mist often to increase humidity. Feed bimonthly with liquid fertilizer during the summer, and use purified room-temperature water if your tap water is alkaline.

Soil and transplanting

Repot young plants in spring and older plants as required, using commercial potting soil.

Grooming

Pinch off the tips to encourage bushiness.

Propagating

Cuttings in spring kept warm and moist. New-growth cuttings work best.

Environment

Mature plants that have grown into small tree-like structures work best as regal specimens, although all sizes and ages are attractive. Work well in a terrarium or dish garden because of the ability to maintain high humidity.

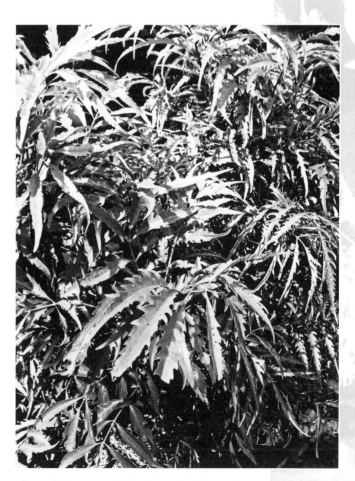

HERDA

Miracle Tree *Moringa stenopetala*

Habit

Have an upright habit, growing slowly to 4 feet or more. Unlike other varieties of moringa from India, these grow shorter with denser crowns and are well-suited to container growing.

Flowering

Rarely indoors.

Light and temperature

These natives of the tropics prefer bright indirect light to full sun. Do well in average room temperatures above 65°F.

Watering and feeding

Keep plants moist but not saturated; mist often to increase humidity. Feed bimonthly with liquid fertilizer at half the recommended rate during the summer, and use purified room-temperature water if your tap water is alkaline.

Soil and transplanting

Repot young plants in spring and older plants as required, using commercial potting soil enhanced with peat or leaf mold.

Grooming

Pinch off the tips to encourage bushiness.

Propagating

From seeds or cuttings taken in spring.

Environment

Plants are prized for their high-protein leaves, rich concentration of minerals and vitamins, and heavy complement of antioxidants! Leaves, blooms, seeds, and immature seedpods (called "drumsticks") are all edible; seeds are also a source of high-quality oil. Do not eat roots, which are considered poisonous.

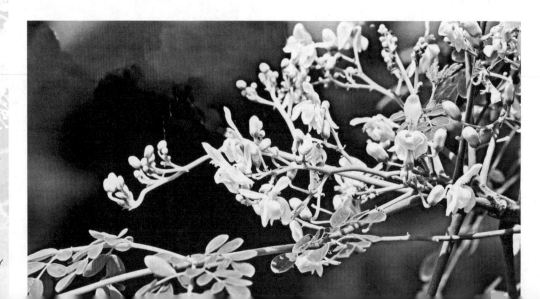

Mistletoe Fig *Ficus deltoidea*

Habit
Slow-growing airy member of the Ficus family reaching 5 to 7 feet indoors.

Flowering
None visible.

Light and temperature
Prefer good indirect light and 70° to 80°F temperatures in summer, down to 65°F in winter.

Watering and feeding
Like moist (not saturated) soil so water accordingly 1 or 2 times a week. Cut back in winter. Feed bimonthly.

Soil and transplanting
Do well in commercial potting soil. Repot young plants yearly in spring and older plants as required.

Grooming
Best if headed back to desired height and allowed to grow like a shrub as opposed to a tree.

Propagating
Cuttings from thin woody shoots in summer.

Environment
Look best as a solo specimen or when set near shorter spiky plants, such as palm grass. The berries common to all fig trees contrast nicely with the attractive round leaves.

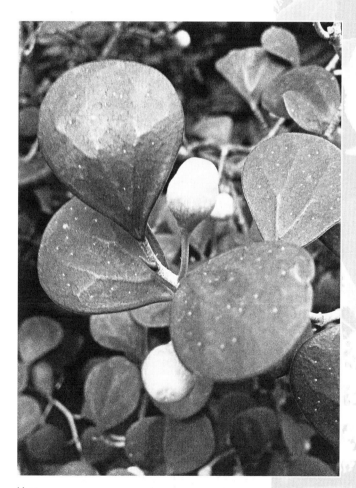

HERDA

Mock Orange *Pitosporum tobira 'Variegata'*

Habit

Grow to 3 to 4 feet in containers and boast attractive glossy, leathery leaves circling the tips of the shoots. Evergreen, the showiest varieties are the 'Variegata," featuring white highlights across the green leaves.

Flowering

Bloom for one week or so in spring or summer with clusters of creamy-white flowers similar to orange blossoms and having an orange-like fragrance, accounting for this plant's name.

Watering and feeding

Water regularly through the growing season and more sparingly in winter. Feed with liquid fertilizer bimonthly during summer.

Soil and transplanting

Grow well in commercial potting soil mixed with sand to provide for greater drainage. Repot in spring as required.

Grooming

Can be headed back in spring to control growth and maintain shape.

Propagating

By cuttings or seed.

Environment

These fast-growing plants do well in bright indirect light for best foliage production.

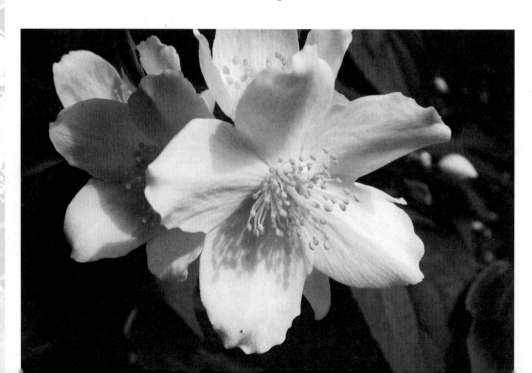

Money Tree *Pachira aquatica*

Habit

These plants are the perfect addition to an interior requiring a tropical feel. Often purchased with multiple trunks braided together.

Flowering

Rarely indoors.

Light and temperature

Thrive in full sun to partial shade, making these sturdy trees excellent candidates for growing in offices and under artificial lighting. Avoid temperatures below 60°F.

Watering and feeding

Require thorough drenching, allowing the soil to dry out between waterings. Apply liquid food at half the recommended dosage bimonthly.

Soil and transplanting

Repot in early spring every 2 years or as required, using rich humus or clean peat.

Grooming

Remove dead leaves and branches.

Propagating

From seeds or cuttings taken in spring.

Environment

These stately evergreen trees do well in containers and tolerate a wide range of lighting conditions. Provide moisture by daily misting. Avoid moving around too often, or the trees will respond with a loss of some leaves.

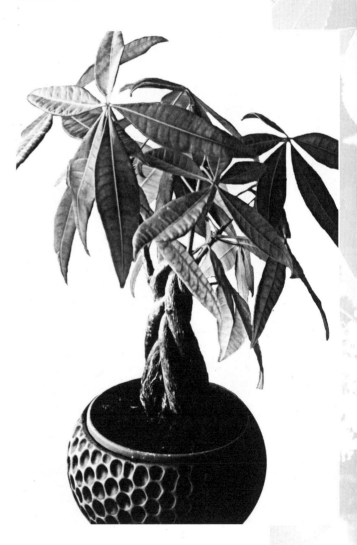

PIXABAY

Neem Tree *Azadirachta indica*

Habit

These hardy trees can tolerate temperatures from 35°F to 120°F, although extended cool weather will cause them to drop their leaves. If you can locate fresh neem tree seeds, you can grow and train this attractive tree indoors.

Flowering

Attractive small clusters of white blossoms resembling those of an orange tree.

Light and temperature

Prefer a well-lighted location but not direct sun, which could cause browning out

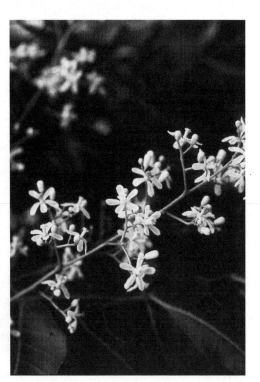

and serious damage over time. Do well in normal room temperatures.

Watering and feeding

Water thoroughly once a week throughout growing season, but avoid saturated soil. Cut back on watering during winter. Feed bimonthly throughout the growing season, and stop feeding during winter.

Soil and transplanting

Do well in nutrient-dense soil with plenty of perlite to encourage drainage and oxygen for the roots. Repot when necessary in early spring before the plants begin new growth.

Grooming

Require grooming only for maintenance when the lower branches lose needles. Cut dried branches back to the trunk.

Propagating

Propagate from seed or cuttings.

Environment

Grow well as single specimens and create a lush green, tropical feel to any room they inhabit. Grow well in east- and north-facing windows.

PEDRO ACEVEDO-RODRIGUEZ, HOSTED BY THE *USDA-NRCS PLANTS DATABASE*

Norfolk Island Pine *Araucaria heterophylla*

Habit

These slow-growing, exotic-looking evergreen trees rarely exceed 6 or 7 feet indoors, producing approximately one new tier of horizontal branches each year.

Flowering

None.

Light and temperature

Prefer a well-lighted location without direct sun, which could cause browning out and needle-drop. Grow well in average house temperatures and can tolerate as low as 50°F in winter.

Watering and feeding

Water thoroughly once a week through-out growing season, and cut back during winter. Feed every 2 weeks. Growing season may be extended to year-round by maintaining high light level during winter.

Soil and transplanting

Nutrient-dense soil includes peat with a little clay, compost, and 25 percent fine sand. Repotting should be done early in spring, before the plant resumes full growth. Repot as required, approximately every 3 to 4 years.

Grooming

Require grooming only for maintenance when the lower branches lose needles. Cut dried branches back to the trunk.

Propagating

Propagate from seed.

Environment

Norfolk Island pines grow well as single specimens or in groups of several trees in the same pot. Small plants do well in a north-facing window.

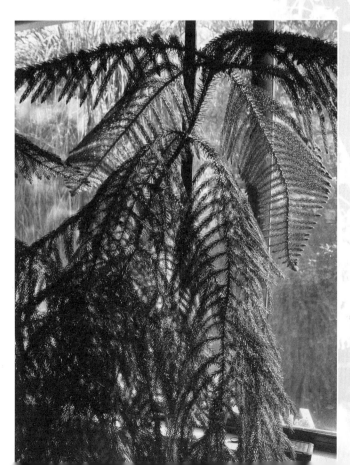

HERDA

North Carolina Cherry *Prunus caroliniana*

Habit

Compact-growing evergreen shrubs that can reach 30 feet outdoors, these handsome glossy-leaved plants adapt well to container culture with periodic pruning. While new growth is upright, older growth tends to be more pendulous.

Flowering

Feature fragrant white flower clusters in spring followed by bright red berries throughout summer and into fall.

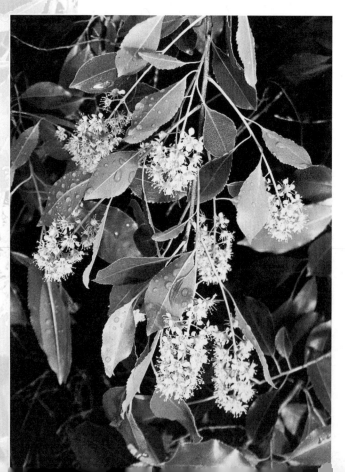

Light and temperature

Prefer strong indirect to lightly screened direct lighting and normal household temperatures.

Watering and feeding

Require watering as topsoil dries out; feed weekly from April through September. Reduce water and eliminate feeding during winter.

Soil and transplanting

Require a rich loamy soil for the best growth, although do well in any commercially prepared soil.

Grooming

Prolific growing shrubs, these tend to send multiple lateral shoots up from the central root mass. Keep side shoots and branches cut back in order to maintain control. When the shrubs have reached the desired height, head back annually, preferably in winter before the sap begins to flow. Aggressive pruning will eventually give you a bushier plant.

Propagating

Easily done by either seed or cuttings.

Environment

A good plant for the patio, greenhouse, or anywhere indoors with good light. Can take short periods of semi-shade if necessary.

Herda

Olive Tree *Olea europaea*

Habit

A compact-growing evergreen indoors, these handsome trees feature opposing leaves that are dark green on top and coolish gray underneath.

Flowering

Feature lightly scented yellow-white flowers in bunches in early spring.

Light and temperature

Provide strong indirect lighting and normal household temperatures.

Watering and feeding

Require frequent watering throughout the growing season and weekly feeding from April through September. Cut down on the water during winter but don't allow to dry out completely.

Soil and transplanting

Require a rich loamy soil for the best growth.

Grooming

A prolific growing tree that's not at all convinced it's not a shrub, this likes to sprout in all directions. Keep side shoots and branches cut back in order to maintain control. When the tree has reached the desired height, head back annually, preferably in winter before the sap begins to flow. Aggressive pruning will eventually give you a tree with a bushy crown.

Propagating

Either by seed or cuttings.

Environment

Good plants for the patio, greenhouse, or glassed-in porch or atrium.

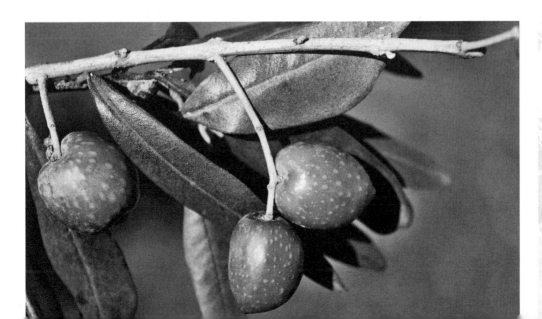

PIXABAY

Ornamental Orange *X citrafortunella mitis*

Habit

A dwarf cultivar, miniature orange trees are shrub-like, growing up to 3 inches a year with proper care to 2 to 4 feet high.

Flowering

Blossom in summer, growth cycles are unpredictable indoors, so they may flower at any time of year instead of only spring time. The flowers are the reward of a well-grown plant. Flowers may be encouraged by exposing trees to a cool dry period (a basement or garage) for a couple of months. The flowers are white and remarkably fragrant.

Light and temperature

Require full sun year-round and grow well on a southern exposed patio or deck. Temperatures should range from 60° to 80°F with good ventilation.

Watering and feeding

Although preferring daily watering throughout the growing season, they can survive some droughts, during which they will shed leaves to reduce evaporation. Reduce watering during winter. Feed every 2 weeks during growing season only. Use only acid-based fertilizers.

Soil and transplanting

Require a heavy soil with some humus and one-quarter sand mixed in. The drainage should be excellent since the roots are susceptible to rot. Crockery shards placed at the bottom of the pot can aid in drainage.

Grooming

Prune back scraggly branches to a new bud and in order to open up the crown and provide for more internal light. Remove yellowing leaves.

Propagating

While all orange trees can be grown from orange seeds, cultivars and hybrids will not bear true from seeds and must be propagated via cuttings.

Environment

Ornamental oranges look best as solitary specimens in a bright sunny place before a south- or west-facing window or on the patio during summer.

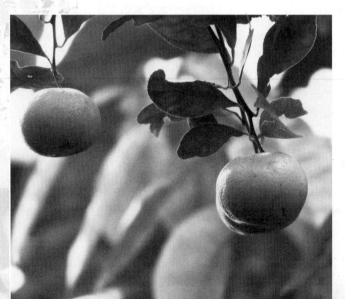

PIXABAY

Palm Grass *Setaria palmifolia*

Habit

Fast growers to 6 to 7 feet when set in a large enough pot.

Flowering

Appear at any time of year on a grass-like seed head. Produce a viable seed that's easy to sow.

Light and temperature

Do well in average room temperatures with bright indirect light to partial shade.

Watering and feeding

Thrive on generous supply of feed and water — as much as you can give it during the growing season. Reduce both in winter.

Soil and transplanting

Appreciate commercial potting soil. Plants do best when grouped together in a large pot. Can be divided in spring or summer and transplanted.

Grooming

Remove faded or browned-out leaves at the base, and cut out spent seed cases after flowering.

Propagating

By seeds or division.

Environment

Need plenty of room and lots of company to look good either as specimens or among other tropical plants.

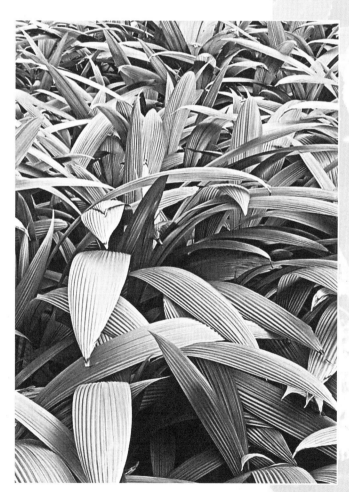

HERDA

Parlor Palm *Chamaedorea elegans*

Habit
These palms are slow growers and, thus, do well in a medium-light atmosphere where they can be kept for years without needing pruning or transplanting.

Flowering
May form insignificant flowers on the side of its stem. These ripen into pea-sized fruit.

Light and temperature
Good low-to-medium-light; plants should be kept out of direct sunlight. Average indoor house temperatures work well, and winter temperatures may go down to 58°F.

Watering and feeding
Require only moderate watering, as do most slow-growing plants. Feed every 2 to 3 weeks during growing season.

Soil and transplanting
Like rich-humus, well-drained slightly alkaline soil. Repot as necessary to maintain balance.

Grooming
Cut off old, dead, unattractive leaves about ½ inch from the stem to create that distinctive "palm look."

Propagating
From side shoots or from seed.

Environment
Most effective as a single specimen or with low-growing ground cover.

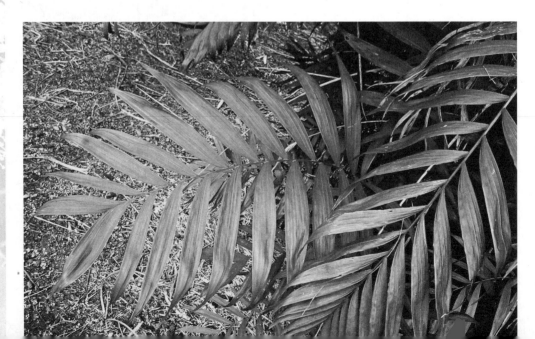

Phoenix Palm *Phoenix canariensis*

Habit

These palms, sometimes known as date palms, are attractive green specimens with delicate fan-shaped leaves. Hardy and easy growing, they are most often sold at around 16 inches high but can grow to more than 7 feet indoors.

Flowering

In good light, may produce groups of flowers at the base of the leaves with inedible fruits to follow.

Light and temperature

Avoid direct exposure for young plants; mature plants can tolerate full sunlight. They can also survive in semi-shade, although their growth won't be as robust. These grow well in normal room temperatures and can survive winter temperatures to 45°F.

Watering and feeding

Water regularly during the growing season, and feed bimonthly. Cut back on water and eliminate fertilizer when dormant.

Soil and transplanting

Should repot young plants in spring, and provide only a top dressing for older plants in larger containers.

Grooming

Remove withered leaves. Brown tips can be snipped off with scissors without damaging the plant.

Propagating

From seeds or, rarely, from root suckers.

Environment

Phoenix palms are very robust plants that grow well in containers both indoors and on a warm patio. Plant either as a single specimen or with other palms for a showier exhibit.

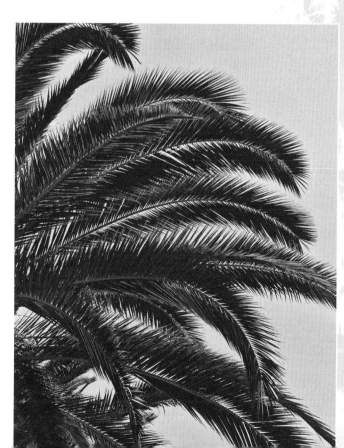

PIXABAY

Pineapple *Ananas comosus 'Variegatus'*

Habit

Although these slow-growing plants reach up to 3 feet high, 'Variegatus' has a more compact form, growing to barely 2 feet. All members of the pineapple family grow wide, sometimes reaching 6 feet across.

Flowering

As with all members of the bromeliad family, once a plant blooms, it begins to die off, leaving often numerous offshoots to replace it. Takes 4 years to bloom and set fruit.

Light and temperature

Need sunshine and warm temperatures year-round. The hybrids grow much more colorful leaves with good light and become pale green with too little exposure. In winter, temperatures should not be below 60°.

Watering and feeding

Require plenty of water so that the soil is always damp. Water the soil and not the heart of the rosette, which could cause plant rot. At greenhouse temperatures, mist with room-temperature water. Feed monthly through the active growing season and abstain from fertilizing during winter dormancy.

Soil and transplanting

Prefer rich soil with excellent drainage. Repotting is seldom necessary, since the parent plant dies off after blooming.

Grooming

Remove damaged or yellowing leaves at the base of the plant.

Propagating

Remove new offshoots when they reach 4 to 5 inches high and repot individually. Keep moist and mist often to provide additional humidity.

Environment

Give these plants plenty of room: their sharp, thorn-like fronds can be painful!

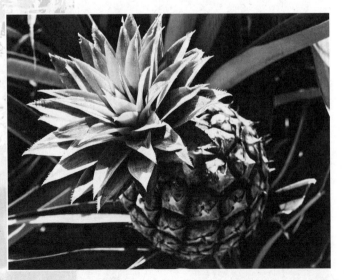

PIXABAY

Pleomele *Dracaena reflexa 'Song of India'*

Habit

Grow to 2 to 3 feet tall, multi-stemmed shrubs. May grow taller and more vine-like in the wild. Unlike most dracaenas, Pleomele sprout new stems from the base of the plant.

Flowering

Rarely produce lightly scented clusters of creamy-white star-shaped flowers.

Light and temperature

Prefer normal indoor temperatures and no direct sun.

Watering and feeding

Allow to dry slightly between waterings and feed monthly with liquid fertilizer.

Soil and transplanting

Provide a commercial mix and good drainage. Repot as required to maintain balance.

Grooming

Older canes tend to vine and may require staking or cutting back to maintain a pleasing shape.

Propagating

By cuttings in spring.

Environment

The colorful 'Song of India' is attractive both as a solitary specimen or near other container plants. Useful because of their better-than-average tolerance of shade.

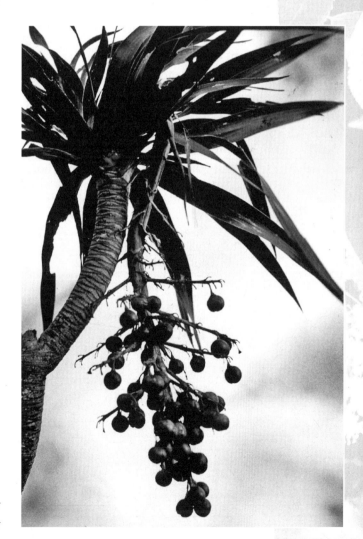

Richard A. Howard, hosted by the USDA-NRCS Plants Database

Ponytail Palm *Beaucarnea recurvata*

Habit

This unique plant — not a palm at all but a succulent — features a swollen stem that grows larger each year. A single rosette of long, narrow, stiff leaves "sprouts" from the top of the plant. May reach 5 feet high or more, but they're very slow growers.

Flowering

None indoors.

Light and temperature

Require good filtered southern exposure and average house temperatures.

Watering and feeding

Like most succulents, these can survive without water for a while, since they hold

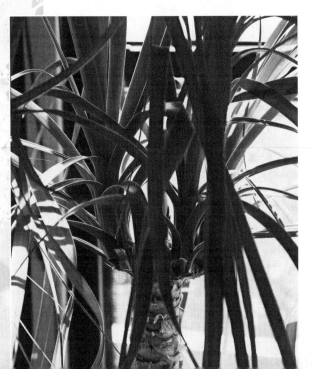

water in their reservoirs — a good enough reason never to overwater these plants. Allow soil to dry out between waterings, and reduce water during dormant season. Feed lightly every 2 months during summer.

Soil and transplanting

Plant in well-draining soil with some gravel or coarse sand mixed in. Annual repotting is not necessary; pot in spring when they outgrow their pots.

Grooming

Remove lower yellow leaves and cut away any brown tips if desired. Also, if you cut the trunk below the leaves (leaving a big ugly, leafless stick stemming from the ground), the plant will respond by throwing out multiple new heads — as many as four or five of them from the top of the stem just below where you made the cut.

Propagating

From seed.

Environment

Work well in any cactus or succulent collection, but they also look good among other foliage plants, particularly palms. The can take up a bit of room since the long arching leaves will eventually reach past the top of pot and down to the floor.

HERDA

Pygmy Date Palm *Phoenix roebelinii*

Habit

Delicate-looking members of the palm family, these make perfect specimens for indoor growth and require little more than minimal maintenance.

Flowering

Rarely indoors.

Light and temperature

Require bright indirect light and average room temperatures during growing season, slightly cooler during dormancy.

Watering and feeding

Water and feed regularly through the summer, allowing the soil to dry out slightly between waterings. Reduce watering in winter.

Soil and transplanting

Prefer rich, well-drained potting soil with some added peat moss and perlite or pumice. Repot young plants every year in spring when roots show through the drain hole. Older larger plants can be top-dressed in spring. Pack the soil tightly when repotting, taking care not to damage the fleshy roots.

Grooming

Remove lower fronds when they begin to turn yellow.

Propagating

By seed or offsets.

Environment

Pygmy date palm are hardy, versatile indoor palms because of their small size. Larger specimens can be dressed up with ground-cover companion plants, while smaller ones make an interesting table centerpiece.

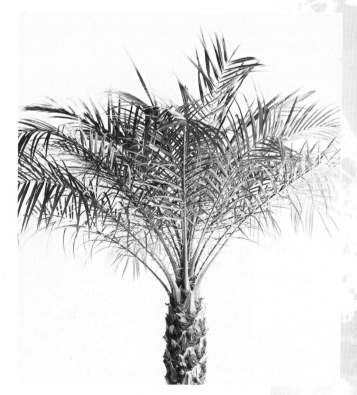

HERDA

Rhododendron *Rhododendron*

Habit

The habits of these slow-growing plants range from spreading to large shrubs or even trees.

Flowering

Flower from spring through summer according to the variety. Blooms are large and showy but without significant fragrance.

Light and temperature

Requirements range from partial shade to full sun, depending upon the variety.

Watering and feeding

Should be kept moist but not wet with good drainage.

Soil and transplanting

Prefer soil with a pH of 5 to 6. These shallow-rooted plants should be repotted about every third year, depending upon growth. They do well in a mix of peat or leaf mold, fir bark, and coarse sand.

Grooming

Prune to prevent leggy growth or to head back after blooming to encourage blooms on old growth the following spring.

Propagating

From seed or semi-woody shoots for cuttings. Don't allow the rooting medium to dry out.

Environment

These acid-loving plants do well with similar companion plants or as solitary specimens.

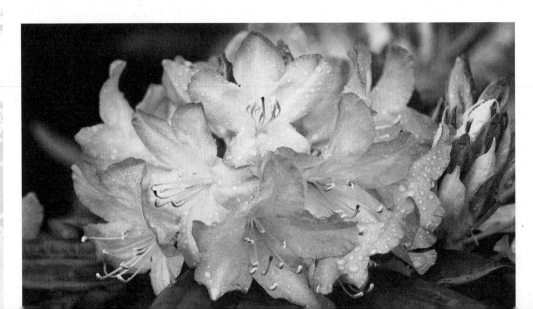

Rosemary *Rosmarinus officinalis*

Habit

Low shrubs usually growing from 1 to 2 feet in containers, these fragrant herbs are evergreen, spreading, and delicious! Can be pruned to desired shape or to keep compact.

Flowering

Rosemary plants produce attractive blue flowers in summer.

Light and temperature

Require high light and average indoor temperatures for best growth. Can tolerate winter temperatures to freezing or slightly below for short periods.

Watering and feeding

Keep well-watered during summer and feed bimonthly, cutting back during dormancy.

Soil and transplanting

Repot in the spring in light rich soil.

Grooming

Pinch off growing tips to keep plants compact, and use the fresh cuttings in cooking or allow to air-dry and store for future use. These make great culinary herbs that can also be trained to grow as a ground cover beneath a large potted tree.

Propagating

From seed in spring or cuttings in spring and fall.

Environment

Rosemary is a good southern-exposure plant that thrives in summer heat.

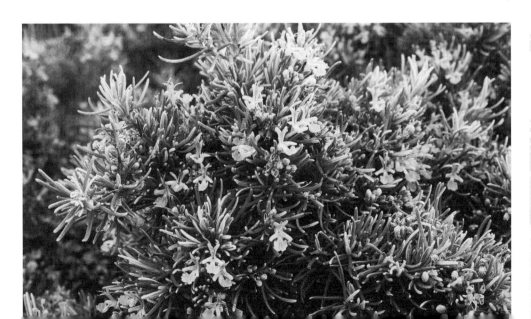

Rubber Tree *Ficus elastica*

Habit

The growth of these tall fast-growing plants can be kept in check by regular heading back and side pruning. Heading back will create more lateral branches.

Flowering

Rarely indoors.

Light and temperature

Require strong indirect light to prevent from losing leaves, particularly the variegated varieties. Average house temperatures suit these plants well, with winter temperatures not lower than 55°F.

Watering and feeding

Large broad-leaved plants such as these required a lot of water — preferably twice a week during summer and just enough to prevent from drying out during the dormant season. Feed with liquid plant food as directed during growing season, but avoid feeding too frequently to prevent excessive growth.

Soil and transplanting

Prefer commercial potting soil with a little extra peat. Transplant into a larger pot when necessary, about every 3 to 4 years.

Grooming

To maintain a compact, symmetrical form, head back as necessary to force lateral branch growth.

Environment

This extremely hardy and versatile plant looks good as both a solitary specimen or in containers with several plants.

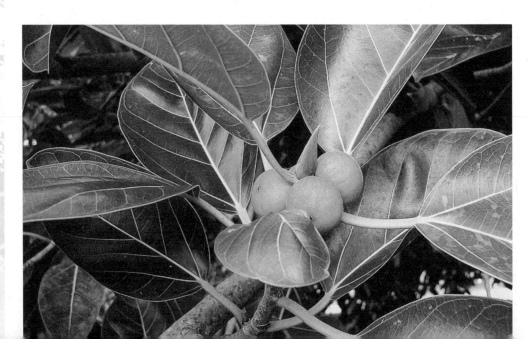

Sago Palm *Cycas revoluta*

Habit

These antiquated palms from a bygone era grow to the height of large trees in the wild, but they're slow-growing plants by nature, making them more manageable but still regal-looking indoor specimens.

Flowering

None.

Light and temperature

Require shady to partly shady conditions in summer and bright light throughout the dormant period. Do best with temperatures in the upper 70s when germinating and slightly lower during summer with winter temperatures no cooler than 60°F.

Watering and feeding

Water liberally and feed regularly when new leaves appear. Mist regularly throughout the growing season. Rinse the fronds in the shower or outdoors with the hose to remove accumulated dust.

Soil and transplanting

Transplant into the next sized pot as required, preferably in spring. Prefer a light, well-draining, sandy mixture.

Grooming

Unsightly old fronds can be cut off, but no other grooming is really recommended.

Propagating

From seed, side shoots, or sections of the trunk.

Environment

Look best as a solitary specimen with plenty of room to prevent crowding. Can also be mixed with low-growing ground cover plants such as baby tears or clover if desired.

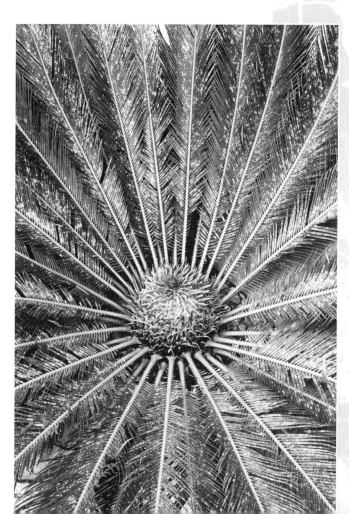

PIXABAY

Screw Pine *Pandanus veitchii*

Habit

Neither a pine nor a palm, which it more closely resembles, these grow to more than 4 feet tall in the wild, although most nursery plants are sold when only 6 to 7 inches. Can grow up to 8 inches a year, depending upon container size and growing conditions.

Flowering

Do not bloom.

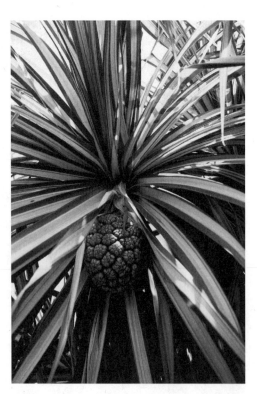

Light and temperature

Prefer a sunny southern exposure, although they can tolerate light shade. Average indoor temperatures and above suit it well. Can't tolerate winter temperatures below around 50°F.

Watering and feeding

Can go for several weeks without watering and even with occasional overwatering. Prefer misting, particularly on hot summer days. Feed monthly through the growing season.

Soil and transplanting

Use a good commercial potting soil and transplant each spring until plant reaches the desired size.

Grooming

Cut away old browned-out leaves to encourage side shoots.

Propagating

Cut small side shoots from mother plant and transplant on their own.

Environment

Easy-care plants that need to be kept alone so as not to prick anyone or anything with their sharp leaves. Specimens make the most vivid impression.

Silk Oak *Grevillea robusta*

Habit
Grow fast, reaching 7 feet high in 3 to 4 years, more in the wild (up to 150 feet).

Flowering
Rarely indoors.

Light and temperature
Grevillea grow best in full sunlight. Prefer normal room temperatures, doing best in the lower 70s. Should not be exposed to less than 45°F.

Watering and feeding
Should be kept evenly moist but not overwatered, and fed monthly during the growing season. Water sparingly and withhold feeding in winter.

Soil and transplanting
Repot young plants yearly in spring and older plants whenever they outgrow their containers. Well-balanced commercial soil is fine.

Grooming
Prune or head back older plants only to maintain desired shape or height.

Propagating
From seed or cuttings.

Environment
Do well with other plants, including companion ground cover. The feather-like leaves make an attractive background for flowing plants.

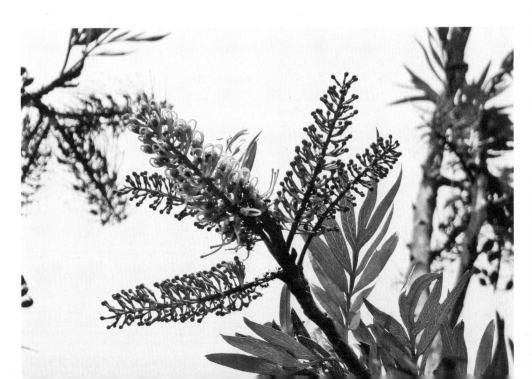

Split-Leaf Philodendron *Monstera deliciosa*

Habit

Named "Monstera" for a reason, these large-leaf spreading plants feature a perpendicular stem and long aerial tendrils to go along with their heart-shaped leathery leaves with holes and deep gashes in them. Fast growers, they can reach 30 feet high in the wild.

Flowering

Rarely indoors.

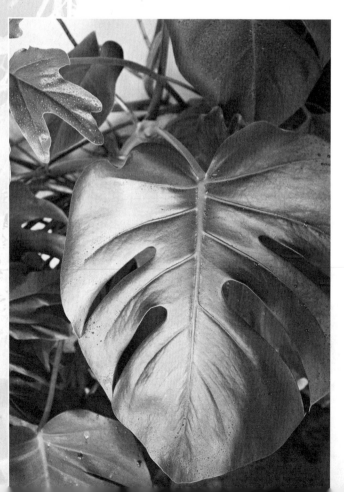

Light and temperature

Prefer good indirect light and comfortable home temperatures and can't tolerate anything lower than 60°F.

Watering and feeding

Like plenty of water in the summer months when days are long but water less in winter. Fertilize monthly during the growing season and stop feeding in winter.

Soil and transplanting

Repot, if necessary, any time of year. Young fast-growing plants may need transplanting in a slightly larger container yearly. Change the topsoil as necessary to prevent it from crusting over.

Grooming

As necessary to keep growth in check.

Propagating

Best done with stem or tip cuttings.

Environment

Create their own sprawling jungle environment in any room in which they're placed. Use as dramatic specimen plants.

HERDA

Ti Plant *Cordyline terminalis*

Habit

Grow to around 4 feet indoors with red-and-green variegated leaves.

Flowering

Grow long branched spikes of pinkish-purple flowers when mature, followed by red berries. Flowers are pleasantly fragrant.

Light and temperature

Need as much light as possible year-long without exposure to direct sunlight in summer, although can tolerate some shade for short periods of time. Do well in normal room temperatures and above. Sensitive to cold, so keep away from doors and leaky windows during winter.

Watering and feeding

Prefer to dry out between waterings, giving oxygen an opportunity to enter the soil, necessary for survival of the roots. Feed lightly with each watering.

Soil and transplanting

Appreciate commercial potting soil with good drainage. Repot young plants each year as required.

Grooming

Trim away older browning leaves.

Propagating

From seeds, cuttings, division, or sections of stem soaked in water and planted once roots have formed.

Environment

Attractive colorful additions to any home in either the variegated or the green varieties.

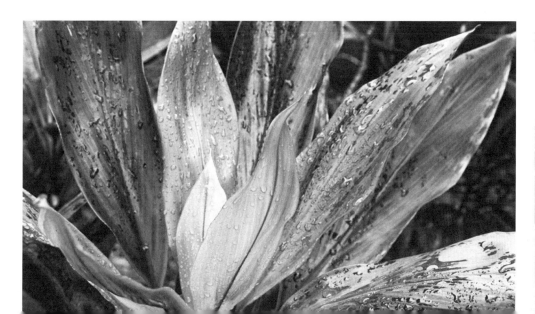

Umbrella Tree *Schefflera actinophylla*

Habit

Glossy deep-green leaves mark these unusually hardy indoor plants that grow to 10 to 12 feet or more, often 3 to 5 feet wide. Rapid growers under ideal conditions.

Flowering

Rarely indoors.

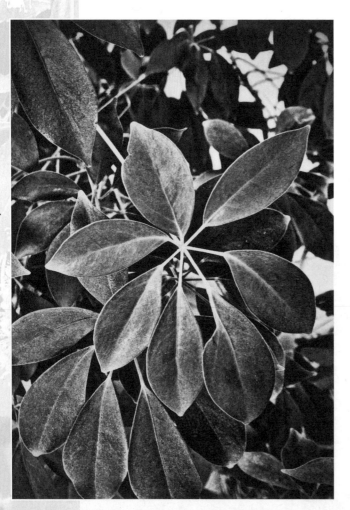

Light and temperature

Tolerate a wide range of temperatures but not below 50°F.

Watering and feeding

Scheffleras need lots of water during the growing season, once or twice weekly. Feed monthly during summer.

Soil and transplanting

Prefer to dry out between waterings; don't let them stand in a tray of water. Commercial potting soil with a bit of sand ensures good drainage. Replant as necessary to maintain healthy growth.

Grooming

Head back in the fall if the plants get too large.

Propagating

From seed or by cuttings planted in a sandy soil mixture and covered until rooted.

Environment

Can be used as a specimen or planted in groups.

Herda

Weeping Fig *Ficus benjamina*

Habit

Fast growers that can reach tree size in a few years, given good growing conditions. Very attractive trunk and canopy when judiciously pruned for the first few years, otherwise they tend to grow into a large shrub.

Flowering

Rarely indoors.

Light and temperature

Grow best in bright indirect or lightly filtered direct light, but can tolerate a darker location for short periods. Best temperatures during growing season are 68°F to 85°F. Keep temperature above 60°F over winter.

Watering and feeding

Require plenty of water during the growing season, but don't allow water to accumulate in the saucer. Appreciate occasional misting and bi-monthly feeding. Eliminate feeding and reduce watering during dormancy.

Soil and transplanting

Appreciate ordinary commercial soil. For larger, more unwieldly specimens, provide top dress when necessary.

Grooming

Remove top shoots regularly if the plant is to remain a particular size, and trim lateral branches and shoots back to the main trunk to maintain a tree-like shape.

Propagating

Use cuttings from top or side shoots in spring.

Environment

Thrive best at constant temperatures, high humidity, and even light. Smaller plants are good for group displays, while larger ones are best as specimens.

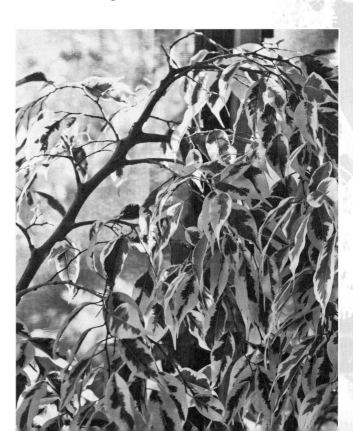

HERDA

Windmill Palm *Trachycarpus fortunei*

Habit

Originally from Asia, these palms feature interesting leaves and fibrous trunks that are used indigenously to provide strands to be woven into rope.

Flowering

Unlikely indoors.

Light and temperature

Require high light, but don't expose young plants to direct sunlight. Can withstand outside temperatures down to 55°F and do well indoors with normal room temperatures.

Watering and feeding

Require filtered watered and food with each watering. Cut back on both during dormancy.

Soil and transplanting

Do well in commercial potting soil or compost with good drainage.

Grooming

Remove withered or dead leaves near the base.

Propagating

By seeds.

Environment

Windmill palms are an attractive addition to any home offering enough bright light and space to spread out.

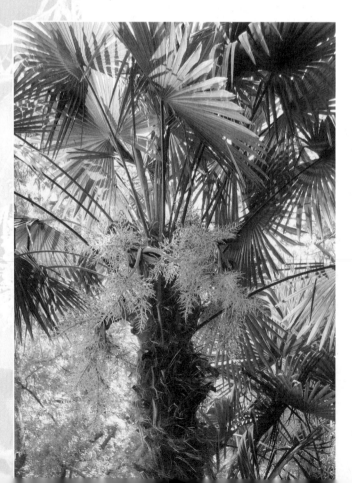

Jeff McMillian, hosted by the
USDA-NRCS Plants Database

Yucca *Yucca elephantipes*

Habit

The height of the yucca depends on the original length of the stem that it is growing from. The rosette of leaves ranges from 20 to 40 inches in diameter and will grow at a rate of 6 to 8 inches per year. The stem will not grow.

Flowering

Rarely flower indoors and has little scent.

Light and temperature

These like a warm sunny place all year-round and need to be watered thoroughly, but then allowed to go nearly dry before rewatering. Never let them stand in water, and don't allow dust to gather on the leaves. It takes away its natural beauty and encourages the proliferation of spider mites in hot, dry weather.

Watering and feeding

Water once or twice a week in the summer, but reduce the amount in the fall and winter. Feed regularly in the summer, but be careful not to give it too high a concentration of fertilizer — ½ strength is plenty.

Grooming

Remove withered leaves.

Propagating

By stem cuttings or top shoots.

Environment

The yucca can be placed in a group of plants, but is equally decorative as a specimen. Since it is possible to have yuccas of varying heights due to the length of the stem, make arrangements with low ground-covering plants beneath. Yuccas look good with such plants as Ficus pumila, the Creeping Fig, Hedera Helix, Ivy, or even Maranta and Philodendron.

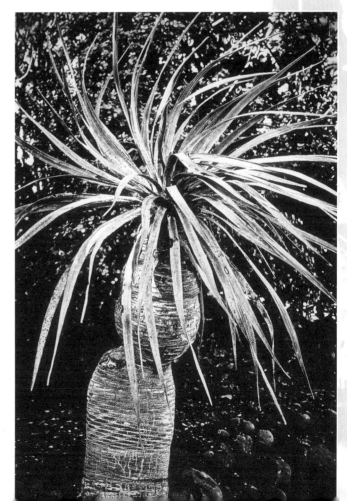

PIXABAY

Endnotes

Preface

1. "Nature's Rx: Green-Time's Effects On ADHD." *Psychology Today.* 2018. Accessed September 13, 2018. https://www.psychologytoday.com/us/blog/mental-wealth/201306/natures-rx-green-times-effects-adhd.

2. "Top 9 Plants That Absorb CO_2 at Night as Well (Best for Indoors)." *Nurserylive Wikipedia*, 2016. Accessed November 29, 2018. https://wiki.nurserylive.com/t/top-9-plants-that-absorb-co2-at-night-as-well-best-for-indoors/315.

3. Long Zhang, Ryan Routsong, and Stuart E. Strand. "Greatly Enhanced Removal of Volatile Organic Carcinogens by a Genetically Modified Houseplant, Pothos Ivy (*Epipremnum Aureum*) Expressing the Mammalian Cytochrome P450 2E1 Gene." *Environmental Science & Technology,* December 19, 2018. https://doi.org/10.1021/acs.est.8b04811.

4. Ibid.

5. Ibid.

Chapter Two

1 "Exposure to Airborne Particles Causes Serious Health Problems." *Medical News Bulletin | Health News and Medical Research*, 2017. Accessed December 7, 2018. https://www.medicalnewsbulletin.com/exposure-airborne-particles-causes-serious-health-problems/.

2. *Tandfonline.com*, 2018. Accessed December 7, 2018. https://www.tandfonline.com/doi/abs/10.1080/00984100290071685?journalCode=uteh20.

3. Joel D. Kaufman, et al. "Association Between Air Pollution and Coronary

Artery Calcification Within Six Metropolitan Areas in the USA (The Multi-Ethnic Study of Atherosclerosis and Air Pollution): A Longitudinal Cohort Study." *The Lancet*, 388 (10045), 2016, pp. 696–704. Elsevier BV. doi:10.1016/s0140-6736(16)00 378-0.

4. "Steel Mill Pollution Linked to Mutations in Study Mice." *Ohiocitizen. org*, 2018. Accessed December 7, 2018. http://www.ohiocitizen.org/ campaigns/aks/study_mice.htm.

5. "NAAQS Table | US EPA." *US EPA*, 2014. Accessed December 7, 2018. https://www.epa.gov/ criteria-air-pollutants/naaqs-table.

6. "The Positive Health Benefits of Negative Ions." *Nutrition Review*, 2013. Accessed April 11, 2019. https:// nutritionreview.org/2013/04/ positive-health-benefits-negative-ions/.

7. Ibid.

8. Ibid.

9. "Negative Ions." 2018. Accessed December 7, 2018. http://mypower bandz.com/what-are-and-what-do-negative-ions-do.html.

10. C. Gubb, T. Blanusa, A. Griffiths, and C. Pfrang. "Can Houseplants Improve Indoor Air Quality by Removing CO_2 and Increasing Relative Humidity?" *Air Quality, Atmosphere & Health*, 2018. Springer Nature America. doi:10.1007/s11869-018-0618-9.

11. "Trinidad, Colorado Health." *Bestplaces.net*, 2019. Accessed April 11, 2019. https://www.bestplaces.net/ health/city/colorado/trinidad.

12. Ibid.

Chapter Three

1. "Can House Plants Reduce Energy Costs?" *Homeguides.sfgate.com*, 2018. Accessed September 17, 2018. https://homeguides.sfgate.com/ can-house-plants-reduce-energy-costs-91627.html.

2. N. Schreck. *10 Ways to Save on Energy Costs This Winter*, 2018. [online] https://money.usnews. com. Available at: https://money. usnews.com/money/blogs/ my-money/2013/11/06/10-ways-to-save-on-energy-costs-this-winter. Accessed December 18, 2018.

3. "Caring for Indoor Plants: Increase the Value of Your Home." *Gihomeloans. com*, 2018. Accessed December 25, 2018. https://gihomeloans.com/ caring-for-indoor-plants-increase-the-value-of-your-home/.

4. "What Plants Contribute to Interior Design." 2016. *Timber Press*. Accessed December 25, 2018. http://www. timberpress.com/blog/2016/05/what-plants-contribute-to-interior-design/.

5. Ibid.

6. "Short-Term Stress Can Affect Learning and Memory." *Sciencedaily,* 2019. Accessed April 11, 2019. https://www.sciencedaily.com/releases/2008/03/080311182434.htm.

7. "Nature's Rx: Green-Time's Effects on ADHD." *Psychology Today,* 2013. Accessed April 11 2019. https://www.psychologytoday.com/us/blog/mental-wealth/201306/natures-rx-green-times-effects-adhd.

8. "6 Unexpected Health Benefits of Gardening." *Eartheasy Guides & Articles,* 2019. Accessed April 11, 2019. https://learn.eartheasy.com/articles/6-unexpected-health-benefits-of-gardening/.

9. "Study Linking Beneficial Bacteria to Mental Health Makes Top 10 List for Brain Research." *CU Boulder Today,* 2017. Accessed April 11, 2019. https://www.colorado.edu/today/2017/01/05/study-linking-beneficial-bacteria-mental-health-makes-top-10-list-brain-research.

Chapter Four

1. Susan Fiscarelli. "Improve Office Morale and Productivity with Indoor Plants." *Interiorofficeplants.com,* 2019. Accessed April 11, 2019. http://www.interiorofficeplants.com/http:/www.interiorofficeplants.com/improve-office-morale-and-productivity-with-indoor-plants-2/.

2. *Ngia.com.au,* 2018. Accessed September 12, 2018. https://www.ngia.com.au/Attachment?Action=Download&Attachment_id=1430.

3. Shiv Malik. "Plants in Offices Increase Happiness and Productivity." *The Guardian,* August 13, 2014. Accessed September 12, 2018. https://www.theguardian.com/money/2014/aug/31/plants-offices-workers-productive-minimalist-employees.

4. "Global Study Connects Levels of Employee Productivity and Well Being to Office Design." *Prnewswire.com,* March 31, 2015. Accessed September 12, 2018. https://www.prnewswire.com/news-releases/global-study-connects-levels-of-employee-productivity-and-well-being-to-office-design-300058034.html.

5. Tøve Fjeld, Bo Veiersted, Leiv Sandvik, Geir Riise, and Finn Levy. "The Effect of Indoor Foliage Plants on Health and Discomfort Symptoms Among Office Workers." *Indoor and Built Environment,* July 1, 1998. http://journals.sagepub.com/doi/abs/10.1177/1420326X9800700404?ssource=mfc&rss=1&.

6. Tøve Fjeld. "Benefits of Office Plants." *Ieqindoorplants.com.au,* May 13, 2018. Accessed September 12, 2018.

https://www.ieqindoorplants.com.au/benefits-of-office-plants/.

7. "Global Study." Accessed September 12, 2018.

8. P. Costa and R.W. James. "Constructive Use of Vegetation in Office Buildings." Presented at the Plants for People Symposium, November 23, 1995 at the Hague, Holland. *Greenplantsforgreenbuildings.org*. Accessed September 12, 2018. https://greenplantsforgreenbuildings.org/wp-content/uploads/2014/09/Silence-of-the-Palms_Costa1.pdf.

9. "Global Study."

10. Marlon Nieuwenhuis, Craig Knight, Tom Postmes, and S. Alexander Haslam. *Journal of Experimental Psychology: Applied,* Vol. 20(3), July 28, 2014, pp. 199-214.

11. Shiv Malik, 2014.

12. Ibid.

13. Ibid.

Chapter Six

1. "Soil and Plant Nutrition: A Gardener's Perspective." *Cooperative Extension: Garden & Yard.* University of Maine Cooperative Extension, 2018. Accessed September 24, 2018. https://extension.umaine.edu/gardening/manual/soils/soil-and-plant-nutrition/.

2. "18. Plants Grown in Containers." NC State Extension Publications. *Content.*

ces.ncsu.edu, 2018. Accessed October 30, 2018. https://content.ces.ncsu.edu/extension-gardener-handbook/18-plants-grown-in-containers#section_heading_8768.

3. Ibid.

Chapter Eight

1. "How to Use Mirrors to Increase the Sunlight in Your Home." *Homeguides.sfgate.com*, 2018. Accessed December 25, 2018. https://homeguides.sfgate.com/use-mirrors-increase-sunlight-home-48809.html.

Chapter Ten

1. "Pesticide Reregistration Status | Pesticides | US EPA." *Archive.epa.gov,* 2018. Accessed November 3, 2018. https://archive.epa.gov/pesticides/reregistration/web/html/status_page_m.html.

2. "WHO | The WHO Recommended Classification of Pesticides by Hazard." *Who.int*, 2018. Accessed November 3, 2018. http://www.who.int/ipcs/publications/pesticides_hazard/en/.

3. "Untitled Document." *Web.archive.org*, 2018. Accessed November 3, 2018. https://web.archive.org/web/20100111030314/http://www.epa.gov/opprd001/rup/rup6mols.htm.

4. "Food Grade Diatomaceous Earth: Human Use Information."

Wolfcreekranchorganics.com, 2018. Accessed October 26, 2018. http://wolfcreek ranchorganics.com/library/de_human.html.

5. "Signs and Symptoms of Plant Disease: Is It Fungal, Viral or Bacterial?" *MSU Extension*, 2018. Accessed October 26, 2018. https://www.canr.msu.edu/news/signs_and_symptoms_of_plant_disease_is_it_fungal_viral_or_bacterial.

6. "Bacterial and Fungal Leaf Spot." *Planet Natural*. www.planetnatural.com/pest-problem-solver/plant-disease/bacterial-leaf-spot/. Accessed October 27, 2018.

7. "Plant Diseases: Identification & Control." *Planet Natural*. www.planetnatural.com/pest-problem-solver/plant-disease/.

8. "Organic Fungicides." *Planet Natural*. www.planetnatural.com/product-category/natural-pest-control/fungicides-plant-disease/. Accessed October 27, 2018.

Chapter Eleven

1. Montague Free. *Plant Propagation in Pictures.* New York: Doubleday, 1957.

2. "Plant Propagation by Stem Cuttings." *Content.ces.ncsu.edu,* 2018. Accessed September 28, 2018. https://content.ces.ncsu.edu/plant-propagation-by-stem-cuttings-instructions-for-the-home-gardener.

3. Ibid.

4. Ibid.

5. Ibid.

Chapter Twelve

1. Jeffrey Williamson. "HS57/MG243: Growing Fruit Crops in Containers." *Edis.ifas.ufl.edu*, 2018. Accessed September 29, 2018. http://edis.ifas.ufl.edu/mg243.

Chapter Thirteen

1. "Growdiaries. Top 10 of Tiny Marijuana Varieties." *Greenparrotseeds.com*, 2018. Accessed October 27, 2018. https://greenparrotseeds.com/en/blog/107-top-10-of-tiny-marijuana-varieties.

2. "Baby Cakes™ Blackberry." *Monrovia.com*, 2018. Accessed October 27, 2018. https://www.monrovia.com/plant-catalog/plants/5486/baby-cakes-blackberry/.

3. "Wild Quinine, *Parthenium integrifolium*, Missouri Snakeroot, Herb Uses and Pictures." *Altnature.com,* 2018. Accessed September 17, 2018. https://altnature.com/gallery/wildquinine.htm.

4. "Burdock: The Annoying Weed That Can Save Your Life." *Ask A Prepper,* 2015. Accessed September 17, 2018.

5. Altnature.com. *Burdock Herb,* 2018. [online] https://altnature.com/gallery/burdock.htm Accessed September 17, 2018].

6. "Plantain Herb Facts and Health Benefits." *Healthbenefitstimes.com,* 2018. Accessed December 27, 2018. https://www.healthbenefitstimes.com/plantain-herb/.

7. "Stanford Researchers Find Electrical Current Stemming From Plants". 2019. Stanford University. Accessed December 27, 2018. https://news.stanford.edu/news/2010/april/electric-current-plants-041310.html.

8. "List of Companion Plants." *En.wikipedia.org,* 2018. Accessed September 29, 2018. https://en.wikipedia.org/wiki/List_of_companion_plants.

Chapter Fourteen

1. N. Franklin. "The Art and Science of Pruning." Home & Garden Information Center, Clemson University, South Carolina, 2018. Accessed September 30, 2018. https://hgic.clemson.edu/hot-topic/the-art-and-science-of-pruning/.

2. Ibid.

3. Agricultural and Natural Resources Ventura County, University of California Cooperative Extension. "Pruning Small Trees and Shrubs." *Ceventura.ucanr.edu,* 2018. Accessed September 30, 2018. http://ceventura.ucanr.edu/Environmental_Horticulture/Landscape/Pruning/.

Index

About the Author

DJ HERDA is an accomplished author, award-winning creative writer, photojournalist, videographer, editor, painter, sculptor, public speaker, and college instructor. He has been an indoor and outdoor gardener for more than 50 years, a syndicated newspaper and magazine garden writer and columnist, and a test grower for Rodale Farms, Jackson & Perkins, and others. During its decade-long run, DJ's *Chicago Tribune* column, In Focus, appeared in more than 1,100 newspapers with a combined circulation of nearly 20 million readers. DJ has had over 80 books published and is also a professional mentor and workshop instructor. He presently lives and works in the Rocky Mountains of the southwestern United States. www.djherda.org

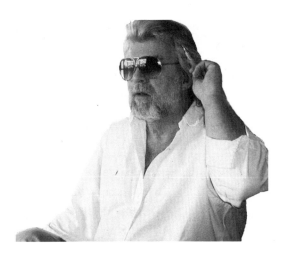

A NOTE ABOUT THE PUBLISHER

New Society Publishers is an activist, solutions-oriented publisher focused on publishing books for a world of change. Our books offer tips, tools, and insights from leading experts in sustainable building, homesteading, climate change, environment, conscientious commerce, renewable energy, and more — positive solutions for troubled times.

We're proud to hold to the highest environmental and social standards of any publisher in North America. This is why some of our books might cost a little more. We think it's worth it!

- We print all our books in North America, never overseas
- All our books are printed on **100% post-consumer recycled paper**, processed chlorine free, with low-VOC vegetable-based inks (since 2002)
- Our corporate structure is an innovative employee shareholder agreement, so we're one-third employee-owned (since 2015)
- We're carbon-neutral (since 2006)
- We're certified as a B Corporation (since 2016)

At New Society Publishers, we care deeply about *what* we publish — but also about *how* we do business.

Download our catalogue at https://newsociety.com/Our-Catalog or for a printed copy please email info@newsocietypub.com or call 1-800-567-6772 ext 111

New Society Publishers
ENVIRONMENTAL BENEFITS STATEMENT

*By Using 100% post-consumer recycled paper vs virgin paper stock,
New Society Publishers saves the following resources:[1] (per every 5,000 copies printed)

32	Trees
2,919	Pounds of Solid Waste
3,212	Gallons of Water
4,189	Kilowatt Hours of Electricity
5,307	Pounds of Greenhouse Gases
23	Pounds of HAPs, VOCs, and AOX Combined
8	Cubic Yards of Landfill Space

[1]Environmental benefits are calculated based on research done by the Environmental Defense Fund and other members of the Paper Task Force who study the environmental impacts of the paper industry.

Certified   MIX

new society
PUBLISHERS
www.newsociety.com